Rethinking Pain

How To Live Well With Chronic Pain

Rethinking Pain

How To Live Well With Chronic Pain

Dr Helena Miranda

Translated from Finnish by Sheryl Hinkkanen
With a Foreword by
Mark Weisberg, PHD ABPP

Hammersmith Health Books
London, UK

First published in Finnish as *Ota Kipu Haltuun* by Otava Kirjapaino in 2016, and updated for the English language edition by Dr H Miranda

First published English in 2019 by Hammersmith Health Books – an imprint of Hammersmith Books Limited
4/4A Bloomsbury Square, London WC1A 2RP, UK
www.hammersmithbooks.co.uk

British Library Cataloguing in Publication Data: A CIP record of this book is available from the British Library.

Print ISBN 978-1-78161-132-6
Ebook ISBN 978-1-78161-133-3

Commissioning editor: Georgina Bentliff
Translated: Sheryl Hinkkanen
Translation edited and anglicised: Hammersmith Books Limited
Designed and typeset: Julie Bennett of Bespoke Publishing Ltd.
Illustrations: Emmi Kyytsönen of Karppi Design
Cover design: Julie Bennett of Bespoke Publishing Ltd
Cover illustration: Emmi Kyytsönen of Karppi Design
Index: Dr Laurence Errington
Production: Helen Whitehorn, Pathmedia Ltd.
Printed and bound: TJ International Ltd, Cornwall, UK

Contents

Foreword

Chronic pain is a major public health problem around the world. Approximately 1.5 billion people worldwide are affected. Pain is the most common reason that people seek medical care. It is estimated that chronic pain affects 20% of the population in the United States and Australia, and up to 43% of the population in the UK. In many countries, healthcare costs for treatment of chronic pain outstrip those of cancer and cardiovascular disease combined. It is one of the leading causes of long-term disability.

Over 75% of patients with chronic pain report feeling depressed due to their pain, and over 50% of chronic pain sufferers feel that they have little or no control over their pain.

And yet, chronic pain is still considered a 'black box' in medicine, shrouded in mystery, confusion, and frustration. It is ubiquitous and poorly understood. Chronic pain represents a complex hologram of biomechanical, neurophysiological, neurohormonal and psychophysiological factors. Well-meaning clinicians often feel stymied in understanding and treating these patients. For this and many other reasons, many shy away from treating chronic pain.

In *Rethinking Pain: How to Live Well with Chronic Pain*, Dr Helena Miranda brings a much-needed roadmap to understanding and treating these challenging conditions. She boils down complex concepts regarding the physiology of chronic pain into user-friendly and accessible information that can help the pain sufferer, as well as their family and friends. She provides a modern, humane and multifaceted guide to understanding pain and its management.

A current buzzword in pain medicine is 'central sensitization'. In other words, ways that the central nervous system can become hypersensitized in chronic pain such that our body's natural alarm systems become distorted. This helps explain, in part, the myriad of symptoms (including digestive distress, multi-site pain, chemical sensitivity, mood fluctuations, and more) that chronic pain sufferers experience. Dr Miranda tackles this concept in straightforward, no-nonsense language that helps the reader make sense of what previously has been so bewildering and tormenting.

Dr Miranda addresses many related concepts that are crucial in helping the chronic pain sufferer get control of their lives. These include the importance of deep sleep, the power of touch, sensible diet and exercise, and the importance of being discerning about where and how to get accurate health information. She provides a sensible guide for evaluating the appropriate use of medications as a bridge to eventual self-care. Also, I greatly appreciate that her work is evidence-based – she lists scientific citations for the topics she covers in each chapter.

A particularly important and often misunderstood notion involves the impact of negative emotions on chronic pain. So many chronic pain sufferers have been through years of going to so many clinics and clinicians trying to get relief. Once they have been through every diagnostic test without significant findings, they may hear that the pain is 'all in your head'. Subsequently, they may understandably feel defensive at any notion that emotions play a role in their pain. Dr Miranda tackles this conundrum skillfully, articulating how unaddressed fear, anger or sadness may serve to further dysregulate the autonomic nervous system and thus worsen real physical pain.

Dr Miranda's biographical details are impressive. She is a physician specialising in occupational medicine in Helsinki, Finland. She has a doctoral degree in pain epidemiology as well as a master's degree in work environmental studies. She has over 40 peer-reviewed publications regarding musculoskeletal pain, its risk factors and effects on work disability. But even more impressive is her personal presence and enthusiasm for pain medicine. I have found her to be passionate in her quest to help patients and families suffering from chronic pain live better and more fully.

Another unique feature of Helena's book is her willingness to share her own personal journey coping with longstanding chronic pain. Patients on the chronic pain journey so often feel isolated and misunderstood. As the reader learns about Helena's personal challenges with pain, they will feel as if someone is finally putting *their* story into words.

Having worked in the field of chronic pain treatment for over 33 years, I deeply appreciate this invaluable resource for patients and their loved ones. I wish it had been available long ago! Dr Miranda is a beacon of hope for the chronic pain sufferer, and this book will help launch the reader on their journey of healing.

Mark B Weisberg, PHD, ABPP
Board Certified Clinical Health Psychologist
Diplomate, American Board of Professional Psychology
Co-author: *Trust Your Gut: Get Lasting Healing from IBS and Other Chronic Digestive Problems Without Drugs*
Minneapolis, Minnesota, USA

Acknowledgement

I would like to thank Darren Newman of Darren Newman Employment Law Ltd, UK, for his advice on employers' obligations under the Equality Act in the UK and on related matters which I have taken into account in Chapter 10, Keep working, and the Appendix. Please note this book is not intended to be a legal guide and should be broadly applicable in any country, not just the UK.

Preface

Dear reader, you have probably been suffering from pain for a long time – for months or even years or decades. Perhaps the reason for your pain has never been discovered, or no effective treatment has been found. You've tried many approaches, taken your share of medication, exercised and rested. You may have had at least one operation. You've fought to be able to keep working and may even have lost this battle to pain. A sense of hopelessness overcomes you at times: won't this ever end? You perhaps feel very much alone with your pain.

This book is meant for you. In the UK, the British Pain Society's most recent survey revealed that around 28 million adults are living with chronic pain; in Europe, around 100 million do; globally, it's about one billion people. You are not alone.

Your pain also affects the people around you: your partner, family members, relatives, friends, colleagues, managers at work, healthcare professionals and other people who come into contact with you as a chronic pain sufferer through their work, including hairdressers, exercise instructors and sales assistants. I've written this book also for people who seek a better understanding of the phenomenon we call 'chronic pain' and want to support pain sufferers in practice.

In my work as a doctor, I have provided care for working-aged people trying to get on with life despite their pain. I've also had a long career conducting scientific research on pain. Research has made tremendous progress in the last 10–15 years, and our understanding of pain has changed. It could even be said that a small-scale scientific revolution has occurred. I don't know of any other common symptom – a symptom affecting everyone – for which new scientific knowledge would have been equally revolutionary.

You're entitled to accurate information about pain and about how you can take care of yourself best. For this book, I've collected together the scattered new scientific knowledge and tried to make it easy to grasp.

All pain is experienced in the brain. To understand this, I'll take you on a short trip through the fascinating world of brain research. It's important to appreciate what happens in the brain when experiencing pain, and what changes prolonged pain causes there.

This book makes its most important contribution at the practical level. I want to provide you with pain management tools that work well and are easy to use – tools that are based on scientific knowledge and that give you the means to feel better. You can start using these tools right away even though the causes of your pain may be unclear and further investigations may be on the horizon.

This book doesn't present the medical criteria for various pain diagnoses, nor does it explain the function of surgical treatments, anaesthetic injections, pain pumps or electronic nerve stimulators. As important as these treatments are to some pain patients, they don't play a decisive role in the management of chronic pain. Your healthcare provider can give you additional information, specific to your situation, about them. You may also wonder why the book contains very little traditional stretching and exercise instruction or advice. That information can be found in existing manuals on pain. In this book, I want to approach things from a new perspective and on the basis of the latest research data.

The book contains 18 chapters, each devoted to a different practical tool for pain management. In each, I tell you about that tool, including how beneficial it can be relative to other approaches, why it works, what the latest research findings tell us about it, my own experience of it both as a pain-physician and as a pain sufferer, how to use it and where to start if you want to learn more about it. After reading this book, you may feel brave enough to begin trying out at least five new tools. I promise you that your life with pain will become easier. When you start to manage your pain, your quality of life will improve and you'll begin to feel better.

I can't promise that your pain will stop. Most likely, it will still be present in your life in some form. Nor should you desperately aspire to have it disappear completely. On the contrary, the less you strive to be pain free, the better you'll begin to manage your pain and the better your life will become. It may be difficult for you to accept this idea right now, but I believe that once you've read this book you'll be more ready to take that on board. The only way to improve your situation is to let go of the wish to get back to your previous, pain-free life. You can attain something far more lasting and meaningful only by giving it up.

In summary, the aim of my book is to help you take control of your pain. You'll have the chance to live a good, high-quality life despite pain. There are many pain management methods that work well.

Before you begin to learn more about those methods/tools, let me introduce you to someone who, like you, has suffered from long-term pain. That person is me. I'd like to share the story of my life with pain. Many aspects of my story may be familiar to you. I myself have suffered from pain for many years, from adolescence to the present day. I've gone through the different stages of chronic pain and the emotions it causes. I've made efforts and become frustrated, and at times I've tired of it all and thrown in the towel.

These experiences, together with scientific knowledge and my work as a physician treating pain patients, have ultimately made me realise what my own pain is all about. Through these insights I have finally started to manage my own symptoms. I can now live a full and meaningful life despite chronic pain.

This book was born out of the wish to share these insights with you, as a fellow pain-sufferer. I hope that you'll have an open mind about my message, that you'll take new knowledge and a new way of thinking on board – and that you'll give yourself the chance to change your life. You can do it!

Helena Miranda
Helsinki, 2019

As you read through this book, tell me about the thoughts that it gives rise to: rethinkingpainbook@gmail.com

Introduction

A new understanding of pain

Your pain, my pain

One of the most important new research findings is the subjectivity of the pain experience. Everyone senses, experiences, understands and interprets pain in a personal way. Each of us has our own pain threshold, sensation of pain and pain tolerance. This individuality that is characteristic of pain poses challenges in terms of treatment, but it does also offer many possibilities because everyone can be directed to find the pain management method best suited to themselves.

Because pain is such a personal experience, no other person – be it a loving partner, parent, co-worker or supervisor – can fully understand *your* pain, no matter how much he or she wants to do so. Nor is healthcare always able to provide adequate understanding and the individual support a pain patient needs. Without doubt, the sincere objective of all healthcare professionals is to alleviate the suffering of a person with pain symptoms, but it just isn't always possible to give enough time, or there isn't always enough information about what the right kinds of support are.

Empathy, listening and empowerment are absolutely central to treating pain. Unfortunately, Western medical training doesn't really teach these skills at all, and traditionally concentrates instead on diagnosing and treating diseases. Medicine diverges and specialises into narrower entities all the time – and this is worrying in terms of pain management. Of issues pertaining to health, pain in particular should be viewed holistically so that the forest can be seen for the trees, as the saying goes. The forest is a human being with not only a body but also a mind and emotions. The trees are the body parts, such as joints, muscles, bones, nerves and cells.

Everyone experiences pain sometimes. It is a perfectly normal part of human life. As a person ages, it is actually quite unusual not to have some aches and pains. Most working-aged people currently have some sort of pain, most often back, neck, head or knee pain. Even young people aren't free of back and neck complaints.

Of course, there are completely pain-free people, too. A circus performer horrifies the audience by sticking long steel needles through his cheeks. He is one of the few thousand people in the world who lack the inborn ability to feel pain. Complete painlessness may sound pleasant, but it is an abnormal and potentially fatal condition caused by a rare genetic defect. These people have a short life expectancy and many of them die at a young age. The cause of death is often an accident or severe infection that spreads because there was no pain to warn them of the danger.

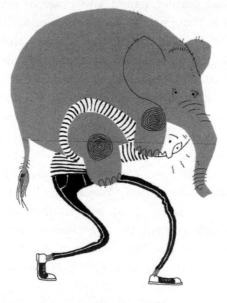

Acute pain thus serves as a warning signal. Pain protects us and teaches us to recognise our limits so that we can avoid injuring ourselves. This role is very important, because in this way pain ultimately sustains life.

When acute pain remains untreated or pain is otherwise prolonged, the pain pathways of the central nervous system may become sensitised to pain, and pain may remain 'on' in the brain. The original trauma causing the pain, such as a foot injury, may heal completely, but the disturbed nerve fibres of the pain pathway continue to tell the brain that the foot hurts. According to current knowledge, any common pain symptom can become chronic and can sensitise the pain pathways of the central nervous system. Typical conditions associated with this phenomenon include back pain, headache, osteoarthritis and rheumatoid arthritis, irritable bowel syndrome and fibromyalgia. A person may simultaneously have, for instance, inflammatory pain caused by rheumatoid arthritis locally in a joint, and more general pain due to sensitisation of the central nervous system and the brain.

Pain that has become chronic and that has at the same time sensitised the central nervous system, is hardly ever a sign of danger, at least not in the same way as acute pain. Chronic pain therefore shouldn't be viewed in the same way as acute pain. I will come back to that.

Learning can lead to problems

Because the pain experience is unique, so are the factors that cause, worsen or ease pain and that affect coping with it. An individual experience of pain is always a complex event that combines physiological reactions, emotional experiences – past, present and future – and expectations. According to current knowledge, a great many factors affect the experience of pain in addition to local tissue damage. Studies reveal quite unexpected connections and factors that you might not have previously been able to associate with pain symptoms. So my wish for you now is this: while you read this book, stop for a moment, now and then, and think about how the ideas I present affect your own pain and the ways you cope with it. Keep an open mind and be curious about new ideas.

On the basis of new knowledge, sensitivity to pain can, for instance, be hereditary. Many pain sufferers report that their father, mother or grandparents had similar pain symptoms: a bad back, rheumatic pains or a hip condition. Heredity is now studied eagerly, but no clear pain genes have been found as yet. Aside from genes and their variants – mutations – of great importance is which genes are turned 'on' and which ones are turned 'off'. The function of genes affecting sensitivity to pain is regulated in part by our environment. The regulation of genes, according to current understanding, can go back to past generations or even skip over generations. It is important to be aware that even if pain is experienced here and now, our history, early life experiences and the environment in which we grew up also affect how we experience pain. More 'interesting observations about this are found in Chapter 4, Don't underestimate the power of touch.

However, learning and the gains derived from our learning probably play a more decisive part in experiencing pain than heredity. We learn pain behaviour from our environment throughout our life. We learn to relate to pain, for instance, according to how Mother reacted to our pain when we fell off our bike as a child, or how our parents or their parents reacted to their own pain. We act according to what we expect and believe will alleviate the pain. When our expectations are realised, the brain reward system is activated and a memory trace is created in our brain.

Memory traces are also created when some function or thought is repeated. This repetition begins to reinforce itself and the function is quickly automated in the brain.

When you practise dance steps, or try out a new song at choir practice, nerve cells begin to learn. In the end, the lesson is learned and the steps or words come automatically, without needing to think about them. Nerve cells also learn when you experience pain. Without noticing it, you may have programmed some pain-related behaviour into your brain's 'hard disk' (to use a computer analogy) that isn't beneficial for you in the long run. You may, for example, have taught yourself to stop everything and lie down to rest every time you feel unpleasant lower-back pain. You may also have been told that pain is a sign of danger and that anything that causes pain should be avoided. You don't question the habit you've adopted unless you learn a new habit to replace it. Caution and avoidance may produce momentary relief, but in the long run they can only maintain the cycle of pain and cause the pain problem to become chronic.

Your back will probably be better if you stay on the move and are active despite the pain. Besides being physically active, there are other lifestyle-related ways to influence your pain. Sleeping enough, avoiding smoking, good stress management, and achieving a suitable weight, are very important factors in terms of pain sensitivity and pain tolerance. Much new scientific knowledge about these has been obtained in the last few years. I promise that this book will bring uncover some new and surprising perspectives.

It's probably comforting to know that it's never too late or too difficult to embrace new approaches to improve pain management. To a person suffering from pain, I can say with confidence that you can learn new tricks as long as you first realise why and how. New insights make it easier to take the bull by the horns. Most of the chronic pain patients that I've encountered in my work say they are ready to do anything to get pain relief. The right attitude is already there; all that's needed is something to initiate the change. I hope that this book will give you these insights and good advice on the journey to a new and more meaningful way to live with pain.

Emotions regulate pain

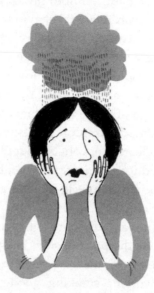

Thoughts, attitudes and feelings have tremendous importance in experiencing pain. Everyone knows that stubbing your big toe on the edge of the dresser in normal circumstances, perhaps when you are a little irritable, provokes cursing (incidentally, profanity has a purpose; it has been proved that cursing helps withstand pain better). When in a truly good mood, you might not necessarily even notice the pain. Feelings of joy and happiness relieve acute pain. Even chronic pain disappears from the mind momentarily when spending an evening with good friends and laughing.

Of all positive emotions, falling in love is perhaps the most effective pain reliever there is. Intense, passionate love starts the brain pumping a true feel-good cocktail of gratification and intimacy hormones – dopamine, serotonin, oxytocin, vasopressin ... – into the body. Falling head over heals in love raises pain tolerance as high as the clouds. Unfortunately, the end of love brings us crashing down to earth painfully. The heart feels tight and aches; longing pierces the chest. (For more about the bliss and pain of love see Chapter 11, Be open to love and affection.)

Emotions affect pain and pain affects emotions. Pain always arouses many feelings in us: annoyance, worry, fear, frustration, insecurity, anxiety, depression. The most important emotion influencing pain is fear. Along with experiences of pain that have aroused fear in the past, we may be conditioned to respond to it in a particular way: we begin to fear the advent of any kind of pain in advance. I'm sure you know someone who always fears the worst. Such a person panics easily and experiences a feeling of helplessness, especially with regard to health-related matters. This feature is known as 'catastrophising'. When fear overtakes our mind we are inclined to panic; the temptation is to act like a rabbit: to hide, to curl up under the covers, to be absolutely silent and motionless. Or there may be an immediate need to seek security and comfort at the doctor's surgery.

Fear is completely human. Our brain is set to fear dangers. However, the settings were made about 100,000 years ago, when survival was an utmost struggle. Then, there was good reason to be afraid. It's problematic that the same settings are still on in the brain, even though sabre-toothed tigers and mammoths became extinct long ago and the other threats of that time – disease, drought, cold – have been tamed by medicines, plumbing and thermal underwear.

For many modern humans, the danger sensors of the central nervous system and the brain are constantly on alert and operate overactively around the clock. Messages interpreted as dangerous flood the cerebral cortex, the part of the brain where the information is processed. Eventually, the flood of information constitutes uncontrolled chaos. Uncontrollable fears turn pain into suffering. In our time, ordinary back pain has become the tiger that may attack unexpectedly from behind the bushes, sinking its sabre teeth into our neck and destroying us, in our imagination. Recognising these unconscious fears and managing them is one of the most central aspects of modern pain management.

Motivation is the driving force

Motivation has a high impact on how we experience and interpret pain and how the feeling of pain affects our functional capacity. Athletes are great examples of motivation. Take, for instance, Finland's top hockey player, Teemu Selänne. On 13 January 2010, in a game against Boston, a hard slap shot hit him in the face, breaking his jaw in three places. It took many hours of surgery to screw three metal plates to his jawbone. The most important game of the season lay ahead, and Teemu was seen on the ice less than three weeks after the fracture. He – once again – scored a goal, and didn't seem to notice any pain during the game. A similar recovery would probably have taken a person without his drive and motivation many weeks longer. A strong will can ward off pain effectively and keep it from reaching consciousness.

It's good to remember that motivation also works in the opposite direction. Examples are found in working life. It may not occur to many people that the atmosphere at work, unfair management, or the monotony of work, can have an impact on pain symptoms and whether the pain sufferer feels able to cope. Sometimes the motivation to recover from pain is reduced because of the eventual return to an unpleasant work community or to disagreeable work following a long sick leave. The experience of pain is intensified then, and so are the negative emotions associated with pain. Pain tolerance is poor, functional capacity doesn't seem to return, and pain is prolonged. This isn't a case of invented or imagined symptoms; rather, pain is a real consequence of the stressful situation.

Today, we are beginning to have a better understanding of the role of work in promoting health instead of seeing work only as something endangering health. Each of us has the right to work and everyone should have a chance to do work that's suitable for them – the kind where they can cope despite pain. Many are excluded from working life too readily because of chronic pain, and that makes them even more physically ill. I look further at this difficult subject in Chapter 10, Keep working.

How prolonged pain affects the sufferer's financial situation is also important. When a person winds up excluded from working life due to pain and their income level collapses, there isn't necessarily enough money any longer for that person to be taken care of. Okay if it's enough to survive on, as many of my pain patients have said. Repeatedly rejected applications for sickness allowance or other disability benefits seldom restore the ability to work; they may only increase bitterness as well as the feeling of being ill used – and of pain. Fighting with the insurance company over accident compensation usually doesn't alleviate pain; on the contrary, it often prolongs suffering. It hurts to be humiliated and there's good reason to lick your wounds for a moment and take stock, but then you should look to the future. Dwelling on feelings of bitterness and mistreatment may in fact prevent rehabilitation from pain. Recognising the facts and moving forward, even if it's necessary at times to crawl, is better than lying down and being exposed to attack for too long.

Our painful society?

Pain is surprisingly culture-bound; indeed, it may surprise you to hear that back pain is a very Western phenomenon. Research has found that Western Europeans have the most back pain in the whole world. Compared with countries with a low standard of living, back pain is twice as common in countries with a high standard of living. The high proportion of older people in the population of Western countries doesn't explain this difference. In wealthy countries, people learn to take note of pain, and normal pain symptoms that are part of life are medicalised more readily. People are taught to be cautious and to protect their precious body. In poorer countries, back pain isn't necessarily paid any heed because many more important dangers threaten health and survival. An interesting German study showed that when Germany was reunified and the borders were opened, the former East German citizens had significantly less back pain and disability than their Western neighbours. Ten years later, the two Germanies had blended permanently and the difference in the amount of back pain had virtually disappeared – Western ways were quickly adopted on the former East German side.

On the other hand, immigrants coming from poorer countries may react strongly to their difficult situation through experiencing pain, seeking healthcare more quickly than usual. The accentuation of pain symptoms in the new country may reflect adaptation problems as well as difficulties in talking about their feelings and the discomfort of their life as a result of language barriers.

Pain is always real

In my practice, my patients with long-term pain often say that an enormous amount of energy is consumed by the feeling that their situation isn't taken seriously. You, too, may have heard the following type of comment: 'I can't believe you are in so much pain when you appear to be in such good health.' You may have experienced that your pain is invalidated and that you aren't believed. This feeling is unfortunately common among people with chronic pain. I'm sure that no one close to you, no co-worker or healthcare professional, has intentionally belittled your pain. What's involved here is a lack of knowledge and understanding, and also a lack of time rather than ill intentions.

Let me now give you some news that should certainly be comforting: the pain people experience is always real. A person genuinely feels the pain he or she claims to be experiencing. Pain is always real.

This fact has been revealed and validated by new brain research methods that can measure pain reactions objectively. This particular revelation has revolutionised our understanding of pain. Functional magnetic resonance imaging (fMRI), among other methods, can be used to identify the areas of the brain

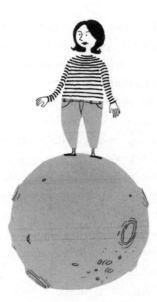

involved in experiencing pain with millimetre precision, and allows us to measure their function in real time. If a person reports feeling severe back pain, the areas of the brain that sense pain are activated widely. Electrical activity and circulation in these areas pick up speed, and the blood supplied to these areas is richer in oxygen, to maintain the accelerated activity. This event can be observed by functional magnetic resonance imaging (fMRI). Brain function and pain reaction can therefore be measured and viewed by computer in the pain laboratory at the same time as the person being examined experiences pain.

The extent of the brain areas with heightened activity corresponds reasonably well to the intensity of perceived pain. In other words, the stronger the pain described by the person is, the more extensive the activated brain areas are. There have also been studies where pain patients connected to the fMRI equipment have watched their own brain on the monitor and, through mental image exercises, have learned to regulate the activity of their brain's pain areas. The person has been asked to think about pain, for instance as a flame whose size can be influenced by his or her own thoughts. Relief from pain, whether back pain or osteoarthritic pain, has been obtained in this way – that is, merely by viewing images of one's own brain. These possible pain treatment methods of the future are exciting! They also give us clues as to what we can do now.

There is thus no reason for outsiders to doubt the experience of pain. This knowledge is also vitally important with regard to healthcare personnel. We can finally move away from the frustration caused by credibility ('The patient can't have so much back pain because the test results and the X-ray were quite normal.') and doubt ('He's here just to get sick leave.'). We can focus our resources on considering why this is the case: why is the patient experiencing such intense pain, what factors affect it and what would provide relief?

The most important of course is that person with pain symptoms first accepts the reality of his or her pain so that the assistance on offer can be received. I often hear a long-term pain sufferer reflecting on whether the pain is only imagined, whether he or she might be going crazy, since tests find nothing wrong and the pain persists. The fact that the regular MRI of the back didn't detect anything that would explain the pain doesn't mean that the pain is not real. The cause of pain may just be elsewhere rather than in the structures or function of the back.

Pain is always in the head

People suffering from pain sometimes write on the internet indignantly, saying that they were offended by a doctor who had hinted that the pain was 'in their head' – in other words, something invented, imagined. Once more, I've got good news for you: there's no longer any reason to be upset. Pain is in the head for all of us. Pain is experienced in the brain, especially in the cerebral cortex. Without the function of the cerebral cortex, we would experience no pain.

The route goes like this:

1. You experience a pain stimulus. For example, a nail scratches your foot.
2. The sensation caused by the stimulus is conveyed as an electric signal from the skin through receptors and nerve fibres in particular to the outermost part of the brain, the cerebral cortex.
3. The sensation is processed in the brain and is quickly given meaning. This important event of assigning meaning is guided by the internal models of the mind called schemas.

Imagine that the hard disk of your brain has a folder called Pain. The folder is a data store that contains your memories of pain, the stories you've heard, the articles you've read, your own experiences, thoughts, beliefs and emotions associated with pain. You constantly update this folder, deleting old, useless information and filing information that is new and important to you. You do this unconsciously. Now, when the nail scratched your foot, your brain, the world's finest computer, started going through the pain folder in milliseconds, selecting a variety of things. In a few seconds the brain feeds into your consciousness a whole made up of the following components: the location and intensity of the pain; the unpleasantness of the pain and other related feelings; the importance of the pain to survival or coping in life, work, the couple relationship; etc. All of the pain you've experienced, whether being scratched by a nail, bitten by a mosquito, or lumbago of the back, is filtered through that folder, or schema.

Through schemas, our brain interprets the original pain stimulus, such as a scratch on the foot by a nail, gives it meaning, and sticks a label on it that reads: Harmless, Suspicious, Dangerous – or some other adjective. On the basis of this label, this meaning, the brain either intensifies or suppresses the stimulus. The scratch on the foot by a nail usually causes only a small surface wound. But what if it has led to more serious

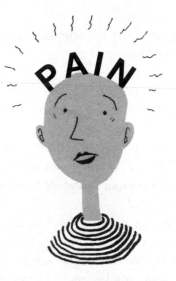

consequences before? The nail then happened to be dirty and rusty, so a minor, seemingly innocent scratch caused serious blood poisoning and hospital treatment.

Now, a new but familiar scratch by a nail, no matter how slight and innocent, is linked with suspicion. Is there danger this time? The pain experienced is distinctly unpleasant. Droplets of sweat begin to rise on the forehead: 'What if I have to go to the hospital and need a drip this time, too...' The pain intensifies and may become unbearable. It is essential to go to the doctor to make sure that all is well. And once you're assured that all is well and your immunisation against tetanus is renewed at the same time, the pain stops immediately. Or, on the other hand, if the reason for a colleague's back pain turns out to be a metastasis of cancer (which is a rare cause of back pain), your own back pain begins to take on new features. The pain becomes stronger, it can no longer be tolerated as before, and you begin to worry and be a little anxious. 'What if my back pain has the same cause?'

Good news once again: because we are able to influence both our thoughts and our own expectations, concerns and fears, we can also edit the content of schemas to make them more realistic and more meaningful. We learn to give symptoms their correct meaning. In order for us to manage our pain better, it is essential that we recognise the impact of past experiences, worries, fears and negative expectations and begin to change them with determination. Only in this way is it possible to cope with long-term pain – and with future new pains.

Chronic pain shapes the brain

The start of the 2000s has been a golden age for research on pain. Studies that make use of brain imaging have opened up completely new perspectives on pain and its treatment. Just by looking at images of the brain, pain researchers can say what kind of pain a person is experiencing – acute or prolonged – with almost 100 per cent accuracy, without even seeing or hearing the person. Certain recognisable changes take place in the brain's links, functions, and structures, and on the basis of these changes it is also possible to predict – already at an early stage of pain – whose pain will become chronic. In other words, just by looking at the brain. Hardly anything can be said about whether pain will become chronic by looking at magnetic images of the knee or the back. (Fortunately, these brain changes can largely be corrected when chronic pain is brought under control.)

Using current methods, it can also be shown how our thoughts, feelings and attitudes alter the activity of neural networks in the central nervous system and bring about measurable physiological changes in our bodies. Thought and feelings are nerve impulses in the brain. The experience of pain is a series of nerve impulses that are processed by our thoughts and feelings, that is, by other nerve impulses. For this reason, it is increasingly difficult to try to separate the human mind from the body, nor is it meaningful any more. As was already known in antiquity, the human being, with his pain and suffering, is a biopsychosocial being.

We can no longer examine pain by just relying on the traditional model where pain is always a sign of danger. The warning signal associated with pain protects the person and life in the acute phase, but when the pain continues, it loses its importance. Any pain at all can become chronic. When it becomes chronic, pain has lasted for months, sometimes years. It may be absent for a while, but it returns again and again. It may be continuous but tolerable so-called 'basic pain' that one learns to live with, but that gets worse from time to time and turns into unbearable pain – often for no particular reason. Worsening of this kind is typical of chronic pain. If the pain is not properly treated and brought under control, there is a danger that one's strength will dissipate, even to the point of collapsing momentarily. Fortunately, however, the pain usually subsides and the quality of life slowly returns.

A prolonged pain symptom can become its own independent illness. I explain this to my patients by saying that when it is prolonged, the pain that had originally been, for instance, in the back moves slowly to the central nervous system and the brain, that it becomes 'centralised'. Although the original tissue damage may have healed – for example, an intervertebral disk prolapse has melted away by itself and no longer presses the sciatic nerve – the nerve pain can still feel the same because the brain incorrectly interprets the signals fed by the nerves as pain. Pain can, as it were, remain 'on' in the brain. Back surgery, ordinary anti-inflammatory drugs, or back muscle exercises are not much use for this sort of pain. Phantom pain is one example of pain produced by the brain: following amputation of the foot below the ankle, most amputees develop pain of the foot – some even severe pain – even though the foot itself no longer exists. That pain, too, is real, even if it is produced by the brain and central nervous system.

The brain plays tricks on us

Studies indicate that nothing can be trusted, especially not one's own brain. As sharp and skilled as the human brain is considered to be, it can still feed us information that is completely wrong. The working of the memory is a good example of this. Studies have shown that our memory is unreliable. Our brain distorts the memory traces linked with the past, feeds new and invented information or information picked up elsewhere in their stead, and provides a memory of the past that doesn't necessarily have anything to do with reality.

A person isn't able to remember past things, such as the pain he or she has experienced previously, with precision. Our memory of the time and strength of our previous pain episode may be completely wrong, and we may even forget having had an operation if we no longer have any complaints. A time span of a year is already too long for us to be able to remember clearly the pain experienced then. Our pain memory depends largely on what the pain situation is at the moment of remembrance. We may even 'remember' another person's pain as our own experience. This doesn't happen intentionally or consciously; it occurs because our brain feeds us incorrect information, a sort of illusory memory. It's offered to us so deftly that we strongly believe that the experience is our own.

This illusory memory trick isn't limited just to our memories; sad to say, it continues at this very moment. Our brain can effectively make us worried and scared without reason. It can give pain a meaning that isn't based on facts. If the back becomes sore as a result of lifting a heavy box, the mind can become worried that the back is now broken. While struggling with pain

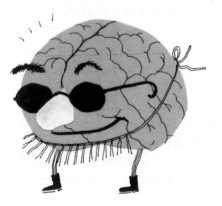

we may begin to fear paralysis and ending up in a wheelchair even though deep down we realise that this concern is unrealistic. Nor is the situation eased any if a co-worker adds fuel to the fire by saying that something similar happened to the sister of his cousin's wife and in the end she was paralysed ...

However, significant tissue damage is very rarely found to be the cause of local lower back pain. The back is strong and doesn't break easily. On the contrary, current knowledge indicates that ordinary local back pain improves best if the back is used normally despite pain.

The mere expectation of pain can cause pain

No smoke without fire, the saying goes, but sometimes smoke alone is enough. New studies have also found that our brain is capable of producing pain-like experiences without an external physical pain stimulus. The mere expectation of a painful event activates the pain areas of the cerebral cortex; a person can then experience pain-like sensations. Just the threat of violence at work may increase workers' pain symptoms. In addition, the pain is felt as stronger because the brain is already sensitised to expect the experiencing of pain, is tuned to the appropriate frequency. The same phenomenon can be observed when we look at pictures of people suffering from pain: the pain areas are activated. When a mother sees her child being injected at the clinic, she also feels discomfort. In other words, pain can be catching, just like emotions – cheerfulness, negativity or depression – can pass from one person to another.

Feelings are intensified in a group. Except in the case of exclusion from the group. There have also been studies where a discriminatory situation has been created in a group of subjects. One of the subjects hasn't been included in the playgroup or a game, and has been left alone outside the group. The same areas of the brain are activated in the subject experiencing discrimination as are activated in the case of physical pain. The subject begins to feel physically uncomfortable, painful. If you wonder how the atmosphere at work can influence workers' pain symptoms, or why the student bullied at school often has a headache, here is some scientific basis.

However, the brain doesn't just vex us, it is also a great resource in treating pain. Our brain can produce appreciable pain relief. This is illustrated best when a person strongly believes in the analgesic effect of some treatment. Then the pain actually subsides. Many of these placebo-related studies have been published in recent years, and the results are astonishing. The mere positive expectation of pain relief can alleviate pain more effectively than morphine. This can be measured objectively through changes in the activity of the brain: the electrical activation of nerves in the pain areas of the brain is suppressed and the person's own pain control system begins to operate effectively. When in turn we believe that no treatment will help us, not even morphine, the pain is not likely to ease up even if morphine were secretly given intravenously (the nocebo effect). Morphine is one of the most powerful analgesic drugs that mankind has been able to develop, but a positive attitude or belief in pain relief is an even more effective remedy. This revolutionary finding should be used more in the treatment of pain.

Chronic pain puts the brain in overdrive

The central nervous system has a complex pain control system that at its best is very effective. Our body constantly sends messages about different sensations to the central nervous system – such as how the soles of the feet feel when standing for a longer period of time. Not all messages reach the brain: more than 70 per cent of these sensations stop at the level of the spinal cord. The brain has much more to do than observe the messages of discomfort coming from the body. These signals are deflected by descending nerve pathways (pathways from the cortical layer to the dorsal parts of the spinal cord) and by neurotransmitters that attenuate the progression of pain signals. The effective 'painkillers' produced by the brain, morphine-like substances such as endorphins, also play a key role by preventing the signal from reaching consciousness.

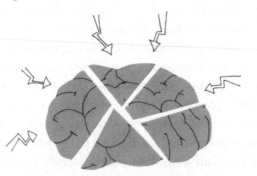

When this system is disturbed, it starts allowing innocent signals to get through, which are then interpreted mistakenly as pain. The protective wall begins to crack. The sensory areas of the cerebral cortex of the brain begin changing shape, and the amount of grey matter in the brain starts decreasing as pain continues for a long time (grey matter is responsible for processing information in the brain). The less grey matter in the brain, the more intense the pain. These changes begin very soon, after even a three-month period of pain.

People with these changes – that is, with a disturbed pain control system – can find it difficult to sit in place for longer periods of time. Sitting for even half an hour starts to produce sensations of pain. This isn't because something would be wrong with their buttocks. Their central nervous system doesn't filter sensations of discomfort adequately; instead, they reach the brain where they are interpreted as pain. A healthy person is well able to sit without pain for several hours straight – although such a sitting spell isn't advisable for other health reasons.

Anxiety and depression further weaken the protective wall of the central nervous system and impair the activity of the descending nerve pathways that block pain. Pain tolerance weakens. These are fortunately often temporary disturbances that are corrected when anxiety, depression and pain are treated.

More permanent disturbances in the pain control system have been observed, for example, among people with headaches, irritable bowel or painful bladder syndrome, or fibromyalgia. According to the current understanding, fibromyalgia is a disorder of the nervous system, a neurological syndrome. Its main symptoms are wide-ranging pains that vary in intensity and location, constant fatigue that isn't alleviated by sleep, reduced stress tolerance, swelling and numbness of the limbs, and sensitivity to draughts and temperature changes.

In fibromyalgia, the accelerating – that is, the sympathetic – regulation of the autonomic nervous system functions so that the nervous system is overactive and irritated. Functional magnetic resonance imaging of the cerebral cortex of a chronic pain sufferer shows continuous hyperactivity of the neural networks. The cerebral cortex is subject to a chaotic flurry of nerve signals. Whereas in the evening the brain should shift to a restful state and people should fall into regenerative sleep, the pain patient's brain doesn't always work that way. It's hard to fall asleep, sleep is fitful, and the amount of deep sleep is slight. No wonder that the person is just as tired in the morning as in the evening – if not more tired.

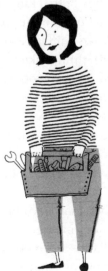

The brain of chronic pain sufferers reacts in a deviant way also to other stimuli in addition to painful stimuli. A person with symptomatic pain can gradually become sensitised to many things: draughts, noise, bright lights, poor indoor air quality, etc. The overactivity of the sympathetic nervous system can stay 'on', creating a vicious circle between pain and overstimulation of the nervous system. The pain management toolbox described in later chapters will help you jump out of this circle.

Instructions for assembling a toolbox

The goal of good pain management is that, as often as possible and for as long as possible, you would be able to enjoy good periods, days or weeks when pain doesn't hinder your life. Then you may not necessarily even notice your basic pain. However, the pain will always worsen from time to time, often for no reason. Then the goal is that the more difficult stage would last as little time as possible, the pain would disrupt as little as possible, and your functional capacity would be at least reasonable.

I speak with my pain patients about a varied toolbox for good pain management. A person with pain symptoms should assemble a personal toolbox of that kind. It should contain many different tools that can be used in appropriate amounts in the appropriate situation. When pain is particularly bad, in addition to medication (if needed), things like a visit to a spa and some pampering, listening to your favourite music, watching the sunset, enjoying a fun movie or even taking a moment longer than usual in the embrace of a loved one, can work extremely well as tools. When the pain is no longer so bad, it's time to take a long walk in the country, forage for blackberries, tend the garden, take a short trip with friends, or maybe try to go to the gym again.

It is good to remember that learning and taking possession of a new pain management method on average takes a couple of months. You should thus be merciful and take your time when getting to know new approaches. You shouldn't give up right away even if it seems that there are no results. Start with the method that seems easiest. Most of the tools don't involve medication. You can also use the tools to enhance the effect of medications taken to treat pain, thus keeping the use of painkillers at a reasonable level.

Everyone has the inborn ability to create health and help him / herself feel better. You haven't lost this ability despite long-term pain. It's important to realise that the pain itself doesn't make life unbearable. What makes life unbearable is the suffering that results from our pain-related thoughts and feelings. The losses associated with pain and the limitations it causes hurt people more than the pain itself. When we face our feelings and change our way of thinking, at the same time we change course towards better health and a better quality of life.

My own story

I'm a medical doctor and a pain researcher, and I've defended a doctoral dissertation on the pain symptoms of working-aged people and their risk factors. I've studied pain for more than 20 years. As my main work nowadays I develop the treatment of pain in occupational health care, and in my doctor's practice I mostly treat pain patients. I myself am a pain patient. Pain has been present in my daily life for a long time. I suffer from migraines, chronic sciatic pain, occasional knee and hip pain, and early osteoarthritis in the small joints of my hands. I've had more than my share of toothaches. As I write this book I am 47 years old.

This is my life: I have a migraine about once a week, sometimes more often. I've lived with migraine since I was 14. Sciatic pain started five years ago. I had surgery to treat it a couple of years ago, but the operation was only partly effective. There is permanent nerve damage to the sciatic nerve in the L5 segment that innervates the right leg, and I walk with a slight limp. The pain is almost constant. Sciatic pain is my so-called 'basic pain'.

I have plenty of other pains as well. The price of my career as a team handball goalkeeper in my youth has been the rapid progression of degeneration of my knees and hips. Some of my fingers no longer straighten properly due to osteoarthritis. The roots of my teeth become infected from time to time because I grind my teeth hard at night and old fillings have begun to leak. And I have plenty of fillings, since I loved sweets as a child!

My work with pain patients is actually made easier by the fact that I can empathise with their pain experiences. I know what it feels like when you can't sleep on either side for more than five minutes without pain. I've also experienced waking up in the early hours of the morning with awful migraine pain, knowing I have an important meeting in the morning.

I'm also familiar with being inspired during a better period to take up physical exercise again, and then finding I have been too eager and started at too high a pace. Bam, the pain sets in immediately after I've started, and is so unbearable that, once again, exercising has to wait for several days. Or weeks. When a patient tells me how hard it is to concentrate when the pain gnaws away at them, I know the feeling: ordinary things take longer, one's memory fails at times, one's nerves are on edge and many things other than pain become irritating – the seemingly never-ending building works in the city where I live and the noise they cause, a heavy cloud of perfume on the bus, the internet being too slow and the glaring sunlight can all be extraordinarily annoying. Arrgh!

When you are sensitised to pain, many ordinary healthcare procedures are worrying in advance: the dentist, electroneuromyography, having a cervical smear test. What if the procedure causes unreasonable pain or the pain remains 'on' for many days? It hurt me the previous time. Do I need yet another root canal treatment? Sigh. Once again I have to ask for a local anaesthetic as soon as I walk in the door, and I must remember to take a painkiller in advance.

Painkillers have become so familiar to me that just seeing the package sometimes causes nausea. I wouldn't want to take any more pills! Still, I can't live without medications. I always carry migraine drugs in my wallet and ibuprofen in my handbag. I never know when I might need them. I've tried various pain threshold medications – and they've been some help. Unfortunately, I've noticed that I've also been sensitised to the side-effects of drugs. (This is common among chronic pain sufferers.) This, combined with my somewhat impatient and demanding nature, has led to my stopping drug treatments too quickly.

I'm a medical professional and a determined producer and avid consumer of research data on pain. For years I've surveyed international science forums and gathered the knowledge on pain that I'm sharing in this book. I read and speak about pain passionately. I've been told that I can talk about pain comprehensibly and inspiringly. I genuinely want to help pain patients.

Still, it's been surprisingly difficult for me to embrace my own message. I've minimised my symptoms, resorted to medical treatment too much, hoped that surgery would improve my back and in the end surrendered to thinking that if I only wait long enough, one day the pain will be gone. I've knowingly exposed myself to work-related stress and I've forgotten to rest. I haven't been able to see myself with the same compassion that comes into play when I care for my own patients. I haven't had time to listen to my own needs as I have been too busy accomplishing goals.

Many years passed in which I lived with sciatic pain that didn't end. It caused much frustration and sorrow. And serious reflection: where am I going with this pain, where would I like to get to and what can I do to help myself?

Slowly – sometimes forcing myself – I have started to test the tools I present in this book. The most difficult thing has been to try medication-free modes of treatment that require some input of one's own. First I had to be convinced by research data. I doubted and hesitated, and eventually persuaded myself to try – and, finally, I was convinced in practice. This process has taken time. But if anything is true, then taking control of one's own pain calls for time – and one needs to give oneself time.

I confess that I've been despondent – and still am at times – and the feeling makes me curl up in pain on the sofa. Sometimes I wish for nothing so much as no longer waking up with the feeling of a red-hot iron spike in my head (a migraine attack), or that the sensation in my right leg would return to what is once was. Logically, I know this isn't going to happen. My present complaints won't be cured; they will always be a part of my life. I've started to accept this also on the emotional level, and this acceptance has been a decisive factor in my life.

It's been a long journey, or at least so it has seemed. Accepting pain has been like a period of mourning, with various stages that just need to be got through. As with grief, prolonged pain brings with it a kind of shock: 'These pains aren't getting any better!' And then a stage of denial: 'This can't be happening to me; up to now I've been so healthy and well-functioning. I'm a doctor. Doctors don't get sick!' Feelings of anger have then floated to the surface: 'Why is it that medicine supposedly isn't able to cure this pain?', as well as bitterness: 'Why is life treating me so badly?' Then I have felt sadness: 'I'm sad because I can no longer play soccer in the yard with my children,' and even some feelings of depression: 'Life with pain is no life at all,' until I moved on to the stage of acceptance: 'Okay, I have these pains. I have to learn to cope with them. Let's get on with it.'

The hardest thing has been accepting the fact that I can't do all the things I used to do before, nor at the same pace. I've always loved running after a ball. I'd love to play badminton, soccer or tennis if my pains would allow. But they no longer do. I don't plan to go downhill skiing or hiking with my active children because I can't do these sports. I'd like to build something with my hands, to renovate an old house or just add a terrace to the cottage. Not with this back. I can't promise a close friend of mine that together we can go sailing for a few days on his boat. As wonderful as it might be to spend time with my friend at sea, the idea of sitting in a sailing boat on a hard bench in a confined space and inclined position, with the wind blowing against my back, brings drops of sweat to my forehead. Ahoy, captain, back pain sighted to the right, migraine to the left – I can't do it!

I look for alternative ways to live a full life – either completely new ways or familiar ways in a slightly modified form. Here's one example: I enjoy travel. I'm a big city person, definitely; I may appreciate the beauty of nature, but I love the smell of asphalt and the rattle of streetcars. I'm blown away by big and bustling cities where people rush around on the streets on weekdays in the same way as people here in a department store during the Black Friday sales. Unfortunately, I'm no longer able to walk greater distances without my sciatic pain becoming unbearable. Just a couple of hours strolling around in a big shopping centre makes my hand rummage in my handbag for a painkiller. I am able to cycle for hours at a leisurely speed without feeling any back pain. I've started to explore cities by bike. I favour cities where it's safe to cycle – and relatively level. One such city in Finland is Tampere, and in Europe, Berlin, Antwerp (a new discovery that I recommend), Vienna, and Copenhagen. I find out in advance where I can rent a bike.

It's been gratifying to see the city opening up before me as a varied, eventful and interesting place – in quite a different way from exploring it on foot or from the window of a tourist bus. In other words, I can still do what I love, but a little differently than before.

I can live with this miserable reality – chronic pain – because

I have slowly started to accept it as part of my life. I can already see hope, light and a happy future in my life even though I'll never be cured of these pains. At least I can still work, but I know that it may not be possible 10 years from now. I've started to prepare for this idea. Nowadays I enjoy my free time because my pain no longer paralyses me. The most important thing is that I'm able to give and receive love because I've learned to love myself, and I no longer blame myself for my pain or for leaving my pain untreated. I've given myself the right to be a person who suffers from chronic pain. I still don't feel sick, and being a pain patient isn't my new identity.

My own experience as a pain patient as well as new research knowledge have helped me to realise something crucial when treating chronic pain patients: I no longer try to solve the patient's problems during one visit. If there were such a solution, my patients would have found it themselves long ago. The pursuit of a quick solution only leads me and my patients to despair and frustration. Today I see my role more and more as an empathetic 'fellow traveller': it's my job to hear and understand people suffering from pain, find out what's involved, provide the right information, guide, support and coach patients to take control of pain. Deep down, the pain patient understands that there's no quick fix that will remove the pain even though the person might secretly hope that the new doctor will provide permanent assistance.

For me personally, the only road to a more meaningful life despite pain has been to get reacquainted with the competent, courageous and skilled person within me, the person I was before the pains began to gain more ground and crush my self-esteem. I have met that person again in peace, listened and understood, nurtured and cherished her. That's why I haven't been steered any longer by despair, anxiety, frustration or bitterness, but rather by tranquillity, confidence in my own abilities and strength, and by the fact that life carries me forward.

Tools For
Pain Management

Chapter 1

Get the right information

Prolonged pain, back pain for example, gives rise to concern and anxiety. Uncertainty about the cause of the pain increases the unpleasantness of the experience. To find out more about their symptoms, many people head first to the internet, scouring it for all possible information – and it is possible to find anything out there, including some incredible stories about the causes of pain. A seemingly matter-of-fact internet site may list all sorts of illnesses that can cause back pain – illnesses that sound ominous to the layman: rheumatism, degeneration, spinal cord stenosis, tumours ... Perhaps the most terrifying alternative is cancer, or even a cancerous metastasis ('secondary' tumour meaning cancer has spread). Concern deepens, and back pain sufferers head quickly for the doctor's surgery to get a thorough examination.

Disappointment sets in when, following examination, the general practitioner doesn't refer the back pain patient for magnetic resonance imaging (MRI) and to see a specialist. Instead, the doctor merely advises the patient to alleviate the pain with a painkiller and get on with life as before. The doctor may even try to reassure the patient that the pain isn't serious. This doesn't dispel the patient's concern, and on top of everything else, causes a feeling of frustration. Returning to the internet to ask other pain sufferers what might be wrong remains the only course of action. Someone will certainly be able to give some advice. But will it be good advice?

The internet provides an easy channel for sharing information, and an outlet for concerns and disappointments. There, neither poor text quality nor inhibitions have much weight. At its best, the internet could be an excellent source of peer support if people whose affairs are in order, who have received help, who are coping and who are satisfied with their life despite pain, also contributed. It could be a great reference and source of help if all of the information distributed there were true and reliable. Unfortunately, this is not the case.

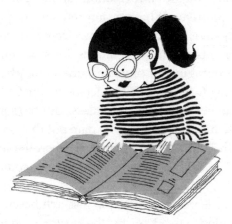

Why a person suffering from pain should seek out accurate information

On the internet, as is often the case with other human interactions, negativity and bad news tend to prevail. In the coffee room, workmates are all ears when a colleague goes into detail about having a handbag snatched or coming down with a stomach bug while on holiday. Few pay much attention when a co-worker gives a detailed description of the pleasant features of the holiday resort. The 10 most awful experiences at the doctor's office circulate among us almost as tradition. The many doctors' visits resulting in a satisfied patient are of no interest to anyone.

There is a natural explanation for this: over the millennia the human brain has become attuned to noticing possible dangers and drawbacks best. This feature has been essential to our survival. The brain works in a much more complex fashion when processing negative as opposed to positive information. We therefore remember negative issues better, and they produce a more powerful mood experience. The brain doesn't focus on joy and remembering the positive; a good feeling fades quickly. The annoyance at losing £50 is much stronger and more persistent than the pleasure of getting £50.

Correct and reliable information about pain is neither negative nor positive. Whether information is perceived as positive or negative, welcome or unwelcome, depends on the recipient's thoughts and interpretations. Information that can be helpful and encouraging for one pain sufferer may be off-putting and discouraging for another. One person is satisfied when back pain is found to be benign and harmless, and he/she is told not only is it fine to move about despite pain but that one should do so, while another may be disappointed when the investigation doesn't reveal a back problem that surgery could eliminate completely.

It's useful to learn how to view research-based knowledge or the information passed on by the doctor without emotion-tinted glasses, whether rose or black. One should receive the information as it is and weigh its impact on one's own life calmly, with an open mind. A doctor who tells you that your back pain doesn't warrant magnetic resonance imaging and that you don't need to be referred to a specialist is unlikely only to be trying to save money, or annoy you. The doctor is saying this because it's in your best interest. At the same time, he/she should assume responsibility for the overall care of your pain and discuss different forms of treatment with you; hopefully a range of methods, not just medication.

Chapter 1

What research tells us

It is important to treat or eliminate the causes of acute pain –
whenever this is possible – in order to prevent pain becoming
prolonged. Sometimes pain persists even if it can be assumed
that the tissue damage causing it, such as a strain, tendonitis or a
fracture, has healed. 'Chronic pain' refers to pain that has lasted
longer than it usually takes for tissue damage to heal (generally
at most three to six months).

Any acute pain at all can become chronic. Such a case may
involve hypersensitivity of the central nervous system, and
what is known as 'central sensitisation' – that is, a pain problem
maintained by the central nervous system (brain and spinal
cord). It has been estimated that one out of three patients with
osteoarthritis or rheumatoid arthritis, and as many as 60 to 70
per cent of back pain patients referred to pain clinics, exhibit
features of central sensitisation in addition to the local cause of
pain. Anti-inflammatory analgesics, opiates and surgery are not
very helpful for this type of pain.

How do you know if your own central nervous system is
hypersensitised to experience pain? This is likely to be the case if
you have experienced a lot of pain throughout your body during
your lifetime. This type of pain may frequently change location
in your body. In addition, its worsening is difficult to predict and
it is not helped by rest. The pain maintained by a hypersensitised
central nervous system doesn't usually begin suddenly; instead
it develops over a longer period of time. Your feelings of pain
may have started when you were young – as a schoolchild or a
young adult. In addition to pain, you may have other symptoms:
fatigue, memory issues and concentration difficulties, sleep
problems, mood problems. Also common is sensitivity to
other stimuli, such as bright light, fluctuations in temperature,
chemicals, odours, noise, polluted indoor air, medications and,
for some, even electromagnetic radiation.

Pain is tolerated better if its cause is clear, such as an attack of gout in a joint of the big toe or a bone fracture in an arm. The pain is then easy to explain, and the cause can even be seen. It isn't as frightening as vague, prolonged pain for which no causal tissue damage can be found. To reduce fear, it is worth making the effort to determine the causes of this sort of pain also and the factors maintaining it. However, the cause won't be found in the tissues of the painful area; instead, the pain may stem, for instance, from excessively intense anxiety about the cause of the pain.

Now I will briefly describe the investigation of pain and also say something about surgical treatment. In most cases of common pain symptoms, such as back, neck, shoulder and knee pain, manual and visual examination are sufficient. Laboratory tests and X-rays are sometimes useful, but they aren't needed very often. Magnetic resonance imaging (MRI) has greatly increased in popularity, but usually isn't necessary for most conventional musculoskeletal pain. People in pain often hope for a scan or special investigations that will provide an answer, but there is the problem that MRI often, by chance, detects changes that aren't the cause of the person's pain but may be interpreted as such.

MRI of the back will reveal some sort of 'finding' in almost anyone over the age of 50, regardless of whether or not the person experiences back pain. Just as the skin becomes wrinkled, the spine shows signs of normal ageing: loss of intervertebral disc height, intervertebral disc prolapse, or intervertebral disc degeneration. MRI can indicate changes in the back even among people in their twenties: one in two has loss of height in at least one intervertebral disc. By no means do all of them experience pain. Among middle-aged people, findings in the shoulder or knee, on average, are seldom 'clean'. It's problematic and even sad when misinterpretation of the findings on an image causes a previously healthy individual who has had a backache from time to time – as most people do – to become a person with a back disorder who starts behaving as such, becoming cautious about their back and restricting movement and normal life. The person's suffering increases because he or she no longer feels healthy.

Chapter 1

MRI is justified if there is good reason to suspect a serious illness or if the pain is very severe, is associated with worsening symptoms of weakness, numbness, or other problems with the legs or if there is a major back injury in the background, fever, bladder problems or a history of cancer. The referring physician should have a clear idea of what's most likely to be causing the pain before the imaging is done. Imaging provides confirmation of the doctor's diagnosis. The doctor must also be able to interpret what the findings mean; which of the findings is / are causing the pain and which aren't. If the image won't affect the treatment in any way, it's usually not worth going for MRI. If surgery is planned, MRI is almost always both useful and necessary.

Surgery is useful for some chronic pain states, but other treatments should be tried first. Chronic pain rarely improves with surgery alone. If in the end it is decided to operate, pain should be treated as effectively as possible *before* surgery – and, of course, afterwards. It's important to remember that surgery is not risk free. In addition to the risk of infection and blood clot, many operations are associated with a new pain risk: studies have shown that as many as 20 to 50 per cent of patients who have had an operation experience a new pain state, either during surgery or soon after it, that may be prolonged.

Also, I should add a few words about the reliability of medical knowledge: like outer space, the internet expands endlessly. Awareness of all sorts of research data, ranging in quality from miserable scribbles to Nobel-prize-level, high-end research, spreads with the speed of a meteorite. In addition, the internet has plenty of anecdotal accounts, tales of experience, perceptions, opinions, beliefs and stories disguised as research findings.

Without detailed knowledge of research, it's generally impossible to tell whether a standalone written piece about health on the internet, or in the media in general, is reliable or not. As with any other topic, this applies to pain. For this book, I have striven to collect knowledge on pain that is as reliable as possible. The studies I refer to are almost all good-quality international ones that have gone through rigorous scientific screening. Most of the knowledge I present is based on systematic literature reviews that have gathered together all the available research knowledge to date. It must be said, though, that there are no comprehensive research summaries available for all of the pain management tools outlined in this book; for some there are only individual studies. For the time being, we must be content with those.

It is unfortunate to have to say this, but the biggest funders of research largely define the topics on which new knowledge is produced and which topics are ignored. Traditionally, there has been much research into the drug treatment of pain. This is largely because the pharmaceutical industry is interested in developing new medicines for treating pain – and in making a lot of money by so doing. For this reason, pharmaceutical companies conduct studies in such a way that the results will help them sell their drugs. And this is a good thing as long as all of the knowledge collected – such as the adverse effects of medications and drug tests that fail to yield the desired results – is made available comprehensively and clearly. It should also be declared whether the researchers who have done the studies have obtained financial benefit from the pharmaceutical company.

Drug-free therapies, especially those labelled 'complementary' or 'alternative', in general do not receive such funding and therefore scientific evidence about them cannot be accumulated to the same extent. Scientific evidence is obtained only for what is studied (in other words, what is financed).

Fortunately, the world has woken up to this distortion. For instance, for the sake of impartiality the National Institutes of Health (NIH), which is under the United States Department of Health, decided some years ago to set up its own public research institute for complementary treatment modes, called the National Center for Complementary and Integrative Health. It provides government funding for several research projects investigating the effects of non-pharmaceutical treatments for pain. The aim of the institute is to increase both the amount and the quality of research on complementary therapies.

There is still much to study on the topic of pain. It's clear that no single medication-free therapy will solve the problems associated with the treatment of pain. The same is true for medicines. Treatment for chronic pain should be as individual as possible and tailored to each person's particular needs. It's necessary to treat the person with pain, not just the pain within the person.

My own experience

It's not easy to be a pain patient and to try to be heard and understood. I know this from my own experience. It's a good idea to prepare for your appointment with your doctor, as such preparation will be of great benefit to both you and the healthcare practitioner. Below, I give some tips on how you can prepare for your visit to a physician so that you can get more out of it.

- When you go to see a doctor and the time allotted to you is only 10 to 15 minutes, focus on your most important concern. Think in advance about what you want to say and ask, what you hope the doctor will do, and how you would like to proceed. Write down your questions and wishes and then present your concerns clearly and concisely.
- If you have several concerns or a more difficult problem – and chronic pain is always a more difficult problem – book a longer consultation. If longer consultations are not available, book a double appointment, if this is possible at your place of treatment (try to negotiate with the receptionist handling appointments). It is impossible for any professional to get to grips with a chronic pain patient's situation in 15 minutes so you may need to have a preliminary consultation and agree to return. Be prepared that on the first visit, the doctor will strive mainly to get an overall picture of the situation. There isn't time for much more even if the consultation lasts an hour!

- When seeing a health professional, the patient often forgets many of the things he or she had intended to ask. It's even easier to forget what your doctor tells you so take notes during the consultation. You can also take another pair of ears to the doctor's with you – someone who can take notes for you.

- Before your appointment, make a note of all the medications you are currently taking, the doses and how long you have been taking them for. Your doctor probably doesn't know which medicine package is blue or which pill is triangular in shape so don't rely on descriptions like that for communication. Also, draw up a brief written summary of previous illnesses, examinations and surgeries. Keep this information in your wallet or handbag, for example, update it as necessary, and give it to any new doctor right away. This will help the doctor to get a picture of your situation.

- Don't expect miracles. In their distress, some people go to many doctors seeking a quick-fix explanation and treatment for their symptoms – and are continually disappointed when these are not forthcoming. Changing doctors frequently generally does you more harm than good. Try to find a doctor (or physiotherapist or other health professional properly trained in the modern treatment of pain) who understands you and your pain. You should strive to create a positive therapeutic relationship and be committed to visiting this person for care. The better the person treating you gets to know you, the more help you will receive. There is hardly ever any 'magic bullet' or miracle drug that will cure chronic pain instantaneously.

- Don't expect the doctor to make all of the decisions for you; instead, show that you're interested in taking care of yourself. Make it clear that you're ready to do your own share to increase your wellbeing. Draw up a care plan together and follow it as closely as possible. If the plan doesn't yield the desired result, draw up a new plan.

- Be honest. You'll get the best help when you're open and say how things really are. The doctor is bound to professional secrecy and won't talk about your concerns to others. Shame keeps people silent, but there's no point in feeling shame about concerns that are part of life. That's a waste of energy. It is very likely that the doctor has heard much worse stories than yours and surely won't be shocked by what you have to say. Speak about the emotions your symptoms cause, too. They may have decisive importance for your wellbeing. You can practise bringing up sensitive issues before your visit to the doctor, for instance by saying them out loud at home in front of a mirror or to your partner.

Here are some questions you may want to ask at the appointment. You can use them to draw up a suitable list for yourself:

- What is the probable cause of my pain?
- Are additional investigations needed? What are they?
- What treatments do you recommend for me?
- Would medications be helpful?
- How soon should the effect of any of these treatments be felt?
- How long should the medication be taken for?
- What kind of side-effects can be expected?
- What sort of interactions can occur with other medications that I'm taking?
- How do I come off the medication later on?
- What do I do if the medication doesn't help?
- What other treatments might help?
- Where can I get them?
- What can I do to manage the pain?
- What can I do to keep the pain from recurring?
- When should I be concerned about worsening of the symptoms, and what should I do then?

At the same time, be prepared to answer questions like those in the next list. (Write your answers down in advance.) If your doctor doesn't ask these questions, volunteer this information on your own initiative.

- When did your pain begin?
- Is it constant?
- Do you have any pain elsewhere?
- Do you have other symptoms?
- How does pain affect your ability to function?
- What are you unable to do because of pain, and what can you do despite it?
- Are you able to move about, and can you cope with movement?
- What sort of physical activity do you do?
- Is your work physically strenuous?
- Do you sit still for long periods of time during the day?
- Does your work involve mentally stressful factors?
- Has the pain affected your sleep?
- Did you sleep well before the pain began/worsened?
- Has the pain affected your mood?
- What was your mood like before the pain began/worsened?
- Do you have worries or fears associated with your pain?
- What treatments and means of your own do you have for managing pain?
- What have you tried and what hasn't been helpful?
- What medications do you take, and have they helped you?
- What medications have you taken in the past? What effects did they have, and what side-effects did you experience?

What you can do

- Many countries, including the UK, have specialised pain clinics in which the pain patient is treated in a multidisciplinary way. However, not all pain patients need to visit a pain clinic; instead, most chronic pain can be treated in a primary healthcare setting. There are many doctors, nurses, physiotherapists, osteopaths, chiropractors and other professionals who are well informed about modern pain management and are able to treat chronic pain comprehensively. Trust the professionals, but use your own judgement as well.

- If you need to ask your doctor for a sick note, or a 'fit note', ask him/her also to suggest adjustments that would allow you to return to work, giving this issue some official backing.
- If surgery is suggested as treatment for your chronic pain, it pays to get a second opinion from a doctor who is well informed about pain. Surgeons, as skilled as they are in their specialty, don't usually treat pain comprehensively. They operate on individual tissues and organs.
- In most countries, psychologists are an underused resource in treating chronic pain, although they can be a great help in pain management if this is an area of special competence for them. Many other non-specialist psychologists also have expertise in, for example, cognitive behavioural therapy (CBT) that has been used successfully in pain management. This approach influences the attitudes and fears that are detrimental with regard to pain.
- I also recommend becoming familiar with the more recent trends in physiotherapy and psychotherapy that involve so-called psychophysical approaches that work on the connection between the body and the mind.
- More up-to-date information about pain beyond the scope of this book can be obtained from the following sources, among others: www.nhs.uk/live-well/healthy-body/ways-to-manage-chronic-pain/ and www.britishpainsociety.org/people-with-pain/. In addition, many patient associations organise lectures and radio podcasts on pain given by experts and open to the public.

Chapter 2

Value your sleep

A pleasant morning, a good night's sleep, and no aches anywhere – at least not yet. Your thinking is clear, your mind is calm. Even the sun is shining!

Everyone with chronic pain knows the effect a good night's sleep has on their sense of wellbeing the following day. Once again, life has meaning; there's hope and a new sense of possibilities. A good night's sleep provides the resources that give one the strength to take better care of oneself. Ensuring one gets a restorative sleep is, in fact, one of the most effective pain management tools.

Even so, many people think that poor sleep is an unavoidable part of living with chronic pain and that sleeplessness is one of the additional costs of a pain problem. When the pain dies down, one's quality of sleep will improve. And because the pain can't be alleviated, one's fate is to get through the night, awake with the pain.

You do not have to accept this belief. The sleep problems of a person with pain symptoms can – and should – be treated effectively and with determination. It may not be possible to alleviate pain unless sleep is treated at the same time. And even though the pain may not be eliminated, better sleep will have a decisive impact on coping with it and on improving alertness and overall quality of life. In treating sleep as well as managing chronic pain, drug-free therapy has an important role. Pharmacotherapy (medication) can be used as support.

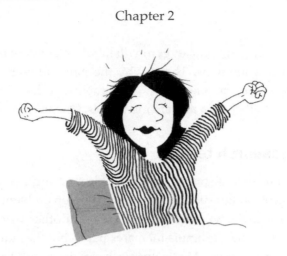

Why you should value your sleep

Sufficiently long, good-quality sleep supports health in many different ways. Thanks to good sleep, the immune system is able to suppress inflammation in the body. Wounds and other types of tissue damage heal better. When a person sleeps well, their metabolism is more efficient and their hormones work steadily. In particular, stress hormones stay in check better despite the gnawing of pain in the background. Thought processes, too, are revitalised when sleeping.

What's more, weight management is easier when one is well rested. A person who is tired is more likely to make impulse purchases of 'treats', and it's harder to resist eating such goodies at home. A person who is tired can't even be bothered to care. However, this isn't merely a question of willpower; it's largely a question of hormones. When a person sleeps well, secretion of the hunger hormone decreases and that of the satiation hormone increases. Balanced hormones facilitate self-control.

Exercise, too, is more appealing when we are rested. Pain patients are repeatedly encouraged to exercise, but are they ever asked whether they have the strength to be physically active? The probable answer is: 'How can I even think about exercise when I've slept badly for weeks and feel like a zombie?' Going to a public swimming pool or gym will hardly seem very tempting under such conditions. That's why the pain sufferer needs to solve their sleep problem first. Only then will they be able to think about other pain management tools. One thing at a time.

What research tells us

Which came first, insomnia or pain? This may surprise you, but many recent studies support the view that sleep problems trigger the vicious circle. So, they both happen – in other words, pain disturbs sleep and insomnia increases pain – but the latter seems to be more common. Many people have sleep problems even before pain surfaces. Insomnia may sensitise the pain pathways of the central nervous system to notice and interpret pain stimuli, or the threat of them, more strongly than usual. New studies show that sleep problems multiply the risk that extensive pain symptoms will surface later in life.

The sleep structure of those suffering from extensive pain problems, such as fibromyalgia, differs from that of others: they wake up during the night more and have less deep, invigorating sleep. A person with fibromyalgia awakens at night on average twice as often as a person who doesn't have this syndrome. It's no wonder then that they experience strong feelings of fatigue during the day. To be sure, sleep problems of this kind are not limited to fibromyalgia. Among others, patients with osteoarthritis have been found to have disturbances in the deeper phases of sleep, i.e., the revitalising sleep, resulting in lighter sleep.

For a chronic pain sufferer, just one bad night increases the sensitivity to pain the next day. The same phenomenon has also been observed among people who are depressed and even among healthy people who don't suffer from pain or depression. Sleeping badly temporarily is directly reflected in the pain symptoms of the next few days. This has been shown by means of questionnaires, diaries and scientific tests performed in a sleep lab. Of course, the increase in pain symptoms affects sleep for the next few nights, but insomnia appears to worsen pain more strongly than pain interferes with sleep.

The natural daily ('circadian') rhythm varies from one person to the next. Half of all adults in the UK are, to a greater or lesser extent, 'early birds', while being a 'night owl' is characteristic of every tenth person. Most of us are neither a pure morning person nor a total owl. A Finnish study published in 2014 showed that being an early riser together with having a regular sleep pattern protects against back pain. Many health problems, including back problems, tend to pile up in night owls. It is difficult to change the internal biological clock completely from night person to early riser. However, night owls do benefit healthwise from attempts to reset the delayed internal biological clock. It can be done with daily exercise, early morning light exposure and regular eating habit. Being a night owl and having an irregular sleep pattern can be part of the reason why some pain management measures don't bring pain adequately under control.

A person sleeps in cycles of about 1.5 hours. During the span of one cycle, a person drifts from a two-staged lighter sleep to two stages of deep, restorative sleep. Then sleep becomes lighter again and, for a short time, there is REM (rapid eye movement) sleep when we dream. After the short REM phase we 'come back to the surface' and become more aware of our environment, before the cycle repeats itself and we drift back into a deeper state of sleep. We do not usually remember the increased awareness, unless we happen to wake up fully. Nor does waking up matter provided we fall asleep again right away.

Deep sleep is a very important stage as the body repairs itself during that time. Growth hormone, among other hormones, is secreted then. In addition, the brain organises memories into 'compartments' during deep sleep, to make room for things newly learned. Problems with memory, concentration and new learning are familiar to a good many chronic pain sufferers. Sleep is of great importance here. After a bad night, it's quite understandable that we don't feel like 'the sharpest pencil in the box'.

Now for the best news in this chapter: with good, restorative sleep, chronic pain symptoms are alleviated over time. This has been shown by many follow-up studies, the longest of them lasting for 15 years. This applies to chronic musculoskeletal pain, tension headaches and migraine. What's more, it's much easier to manage pain when we can sleep well, and our ability to work is maintained better.

I'd also like to emphasise a difficult point that affects many people with chronic pain. The traditional thinking has been that when a person is in pain and sleeps badly, the pain should be taken care of properly so that sleep can improve. In reality, the intensive treatment of pain with strong analgesics, called 'opioids', can further aggravate the sleep problem. Opioids break the structure of sleep, reduce the amount of deep, restorative sleep and disturb the respiratory rhythm while sleeping. The risk of a sleep disorder called sleep apnoea (reducing oxygen levels in the blood and brain) also increases. One out of four people who take opioids regularly suffers from sleep apnoea, often unknowingly. All of these effects further sensitise a person to pain. The vicious circle of pain and fatigue deepens.

These new research findings are so important that I want you to pay particular attention to this point. I know that these opioid painkillers have been prescribed for many chronic pain sufferers who feel that they have benefited from them. Many say that they wouldn't be able to do without them but they do have these negative effects so it is worth considering alternatives. You should discuss this issue with your doctor. I'll talk about pharmaceutical alternatives that are more suitable at the end of this chapter and in Chapter 18, Consider medication.

My own experience

I'm quite a typical chronic pain sufferer: I used to be a good sleeper, but during recent years pain has begun to interfere with my sleep. Neuropathic pain caused by permanent damage in my sciatic nerve has made persistent efforts to interrupt my sleep – and has succeeded. Giving up the pleasure of sleeping on my side is the greatest loss I've had to face. I am not able to lie on either side for more than five minutes. In addition, I find I stir several times during the night owing to leg pain, while I try to find a suitable position to get back to sleep. 'Brain fog' has begun creeping into my mornings and I have episodes when I find it hard to get through the working day, and in the evening have to recover on the sofa. The vicious circle of pain and fatigue has set in.

My wellbeing has been boosted considerably by the simple act of getting a new bed. Although I tell my patients about the importance of a good bed, somehow I hadn't applied that advice to myself.

I calculated one day that my old mattress was over 10 years old. I realised I had spent nearly 25,000 hours in the same bed. As a result, a shallow area in the middle had developed and the whole bed shook when I tossed and turned from one side to the other. I don't know of any other object that I would stubbornly continue to use for seven to eight hours a day even though it should have been taken to the dump a long time ago.

Luckily my new partner nagged me about the poor bed insistently enough that I finally found myself in a furniture shop at the end of a workday. In the shop I tried out two beds. When I flopped onto the second, I felt as if I was in heaven. I lay on my side, which is generally hard for me to do, and in no time, my spine found its place on the viscoelastic mattress. My ever-temperamental sciatic nerve made no objection of any kind. I started to relax and decided to simulate sleep by closing my eyes for a moment. The simulation worked, and I dozed off. When I finally woke up at the gentle prodding of the sales assistant,

I laughed that the test had exceeded all my expectations and quietly went to the cash desk.

Not for a moment have I regretted investing in the bed. My quality of sleep has improved considerably. I wake up less at night. The morning brain fog is now only an occasional guest. The need for painkillers, especially in the middle of the night, has decreased. The mattress certainly isn't the only reason why I've been able to exercise more and take care of myself better than in years, but it has definitely made an important contribution. Whatever the other reasons, this is a positive cycle that I don't wish to break.

What you can do – How to improve your sleep

- Create a peaceful space for yourself with as few distractions as possible where you can sleep. If your spouse snores, ask him or her to move to another room, or try earplugs. With earplugs, the sound of your own circulation may be disturbing at first, but you'll get used to it in a week or two.
- Consider whether you would be better with a soft or hard bed. According to research, a softer bed is preferable, but some swear by a harder bed. There are different kinds of pillows, and they should be varied according to your pain.
- Limit your time in bed to sleeping or love-making only. Read a book or watch TV in the evening, but not in bed, otherwise your brain may receive conflicting messages: is the bed a place to be awake or asleep? The brain must be trained to understand that the bed is for sleeping, not for being awake in.
- If you have trouble falling asleep, stop surfing the internet and updating Facebook before the main evening news. At night, don't check the time using your smartphone. Even a small dose of blue light from electronic devices can be overly stimulating as it reduces the brain's production of melatonin. On the other hand, some people find it relaxing to play computer games in the evening in which case make

sure you have a blue-light filter on your screen.

- A nap during the day may be okay, but always keep it short – less than half an hour. If you wish, have a cup of coffee before you nap. You'll have 20 minutes to sleep before the coffee starts to take effect. For some, however, even one cup of coffee during the day, or at least in the afternoon, may hinder the night's sleep.

- Keep a notebook on your bedside table and, in the evening before you fall asleep, write down any concerns that are worrying you. Tell yourself that your worries will keep in the notebook, that you intend to sleep now and will return to them in the morning. At the same time, recall one or two things from the day for which you are thankful.

- Tell your doctor about your sleep problems. Ask him/her to begin treating your insomnia. Discuss factors affecting sleep and non-pharmaceutical means of treatment together. Your GP or physiotherapist may know of a local sleep group that could provide support.

- Melatonin and pain threshold drugs, such as amitriptyline or the antidepressant mirtazapine in small doses, can safely support the sleep of a person with pain symptoms. Antidepressants or anticonvulsants prescribed for chronic pain also maintain the structure and quality of sleep. Remember always to take melatonin at the same time in the evening. A suitable dose is usually 3–5 mg, but this is very individual.

- Adopt a peaceful attitude to the approaching night. If you start to worry about falling asleep, or if you try too hard, your brain will be stimulated and your sleep is sure to be disturbed. Massage or gentle stroking (you can also stroke yourself!) soothes and relaxes. A warm bath before bedtime, peaceful music, a bowl of porridge and warm socks can have the same effect. Research has shown that relaxation exercises and mindfulness are effective means of improving sleep.

Many small positive things occur in daily life, but they go unnoticed if we are mulling over the past or worrying about the future. The skill of being present (mindful) helps us to see these positive things. It's good to let fresh winds blow on us.

You can try to adopt a more positive way of thinking by applying these examples:

Current way of thinking:	New way of thinking:
I'll never learn this	Let me try again.
This won't work	I can get this to work.
This change is too great	I'll give it a go
I'm too inept to get this done	I've accomplished things before and I'll get this done, too – at my own pace
Other things take too much time for me to be able to take this on	I'll have a look at my use of time to see whether it could be rearranged so that I could do this
I've never done anything like this	Now's my chance to learn something new
Current way of thinking:	New way of thinking:
This is too complicated	I'll proceed one step at a time
I haven't got the strength for this.	Doing this will give me additional strength.

My own experience

I've noticed myself that pain eats away at relaxation and cheerfulness. Part of my playful side has disappeared. I still try to keep humour in my life so I can cope with pain. Self-irony is very helpful. At times I begin laughing at myself and how pain has changed me. Now and then I laugh at my own grannyish clambering up from the floor. Or I laugh at myself when I'm at the airport, leaving for a scientific congress somewhere in the world, headed for the hectic urban throb of a metropolis, with worn health sandals on my feet and my personal pillow tucked under my arm. Today, comfort takes precedence over elegance.

My most important realisation in the face of change has been understanding the need to maintain flexibility of thought. I've learned that it's not worth fighting against pain, but I will fight against an increase in my own negativity and inflexibility to the end. I try to apply every means available so that I don't stiffen up mentally. I look at facts from different angles and I try to snap out of it if my interpretation becomes too coloured by negative emotions. I knowingly break the cycle by turning my thoughts to more positive things. I travel to the Canary Islands, if necessary – in my thoughts, that is. It works surprisingly well.

A concrete spell of laughter helps, too. After having long resisted, I've given in to watching cat videos on the internet. I became enthusiastic about them after reading a study showing that these genuinely do increase the sense of feeling good. I'd previously tried to avoid them, as I'm not even particularly fond of cats; but a few minutes of cat whiskers in action hits the spot. Online series of pictures of funny hair styles and unsuccessful album covers are also effective. I like listening to recordings of Woody Allen and other stand-up comedians through headphones when out for a stroll with the dog. Nor is it a minor issue for me to know that, aside from the calories consumed by walking, 10 to 15 minutes of laughter burns about 50 calories...

I'm quite serious that cheerfulness and laughter could be applied more in our health care and in improving pain management. Everything needn't be so deadly serious. Even among the terminally ill, humour maintains hope. The credibility of health care doesn't disappear even if room is made for more positivity.

What you can do – How to develop a positive attitude

- During the day, stop to listen to yourself and your inner speech. If you find that a negative voice in your mind is commenting on your actions, think how the tone might be made more positive.
- Think which individual factors – for instance, at work or in your relationships with other people – annoy you. Could something be done about them, and could they be made more positive in your mind, one small matter at a time?
- Positive thinking and breaking the negative cycle – for example, in the work community or an online group – requires courage and perseverance. Through your own actions, you can increase balance and bring perspectives other than annoyance into your environment.
- You have strengths. Developing them is easier than learning new skills. Use five minutes in the evening to think about or write down what you did during the day that met with success, as well as the things you're grateful for and a few things about yourself that you like.

Chapter 4

Don't underestimate the power of touch

Why a person suffering from pain benefits from touching and being touched

The healing touch is well known: mother's breath on a scraped knee; a nurse's gentle hug; the hand of one's beloved touching one's arm. Touch – stroking, hugging and caressing – revitalises the body and the mind in many ways. Touch and massage soothe the body, reduce secretion of the stress hormone cortisol, decrease blood pressure and improve stress management. The touch of a loved one or caregiver also alleviates the distress, fear and anxiety associated with pain.

Touching is one of the most natural methods of pain relief at our disposal. It brings people closer together. It helps you learn about the sensations of your mind and body. Touching reinforces a healthy self-image and increases the positive feeling of being in control of your life. It offers a way to show your feelings if it's difficult to talk about them.

What research tells us

The pain relief obtained from touching operates mainly through the nervous system. Nerve fibres located under the skin transmit the sensations of pain and touch to the brain. When the knee hurts and a healthy spot above it is rubbed, this quickly activates

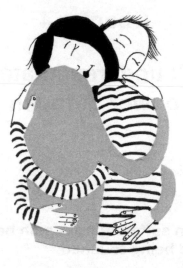

the rapid and thick nerve fibres of those nerves which do not transmit pain signals, called 'non-nociceptive fibres', to carry messages to the central nervous system ahead of those coming from the painful area. In this way they arrive in time to 'close the gate', warding off the slower pain signals leaving from the knee. This classic way to relieve pain is an example of what is called the 'gate control theory'.

Touching and hugging reduce pain also thanks to oxytocin, the 'cuddle hormone'. Oxytocin is a hormone and neurotransmitter that begins to be released from the brain into the bloodstream when a person is touched. For a burst of oxytocin to occur, however, some sort of positive emotional bond is required on the part of the person touched. Massaging the toes of one's partner has an analgesic effect that isn't achieved by a hug at a chance meeting.

Of all the forms of touch, sex is particularly effective in reducing pain. Not only does lovemaking with a person one cares about increase the amount of oxytocin in the body; it also increases the amounts of endorphins and other hormones that produce the sense of feeling good. Nor does good sex always require another person. As Woody Allen put it, masturbation is sex with someone you love. Studies have shown that by fondling herself, a woman can temporarily raise her own pain threshold and tolerance by one and a half times, or even double, the usual threshold. During orgasm, a manifold increase in the secretion of oxytocin takes place and many types of pain are alleviated, including the pain of migraine, one of the worst neurological pains there is.

Lovemaking thus has been proved to be an effective mode of treatment for headaches. Despite this, for many it seems to be more of an obstacle to having sex – in fact, this treatment modality hardly occurs to a person with a headache, but it might be worth trying sometimes. The downside of oxytocin is that its effect is not very long-lasting, usually only some 10s of minutes.

Fibromyalgia patients often tell me that traditional massage isn't good for them; it's too painful. At times, on days when pains are bad, even a hug from one's partner can be painful. Normal physical contact then is unbearable. Yet it would seem that traditional massage can relieve the pain of a person with fibromyalgia, as shown by a systematic review of the research literature that was published in 2014. Massage brought relief from anxiety and even depression. To maintain the effect for a longer time, however, it seems massage therapy should occur over at least five consecutive weeks. Another more recent review suggested that massage, and especially myofascial release, may, in addition to relieving pain, bring functional improvements.

Instead of traditional massage and sports massage, types of massage worth trying by chronic pain sufferers are: light connective tissue massage, tactile stimulation and other gentler methods. High-quality reviews have concluded that there is some evidence of benefit from massage for labour, shoulder, neck, low back, arthritis, postoperative, delayed onset muscle soreness and musculoskeletal pain. Massage and touch, even Reiki therapy, can somewhat relieve pain even in the more difficult conditions, such as cancer. So far there is no convincing scientific evidence on the effectiveness of Reiki or energy treatments in chronic pain, but as an additional means of chronic pain management, they are probably more helpful than harmful from the perspective of wellbeing.

Recent studies indicate that the effects of a lack of affection and nurture, or abuse and neglect, experienced in childhood, can extend into adulthood. Abuse of all kinds moulds the structure and activities of a growing child's brain – for instance, the thickness of the cortex in prefrontal and temporal areas of the brain decreases and the ratio of white matter to grey matter changes, with the amount of grey matter shrinking. The effects of mental or physical abuse can be seen, especially in areas of the brain that are central to stress tolerance and to control of the emotional state.

Similar changes have been observed in adults who later develop chronic pain. The system processing and controlling pain is often disordered. Also, the levels of oxytocin and its effects in the body are different among people who have been abused from among those who haven't had such experiences. Because of these negative childhood experiences, in adulthood cells age more quickly, so wounds and tissue damage don't heal as well as is usually the case. The experiences of childhood and youth may thus affect an adult's pain symptoms in various ways.

Sometimes the effect may be derived from even further in the past. The field of genetics called epigenetics has presented some interesting new angles on both the modern world and our past. Certain events in life, or factors in our environment – such as lack of nutrition or a traumatic experience – can change the function of our genes, in practice affecting which genes are 'on' and which are 'off'. Gene structure itself does not change. Such epigenetic changes can even be handed down from one generation to another, and can thus be reflected in our actions and our health even if the root cause of the change is no longer present in our environment.

In this way, the experiences of our grandparents and their parents may be handed down from one generation to the next, or even skip over several generations. Famine has been studied a great deal in this context. It has been noted that the grandchildren and great-grandchildren of people who have lived in a time of famine are born underweight more often, even if the expectant mother herself has not experienced malnutrition. The change that occurred in the expression of the grandparents' genes, which switched their bodily functions to conservation mode, surfaces a generation or two in the future. It is thus possible that the pain and suffering experienced in one's own family can be handed down to future generations by altering the function of genes associated with the perception of pain and sensitivity to pain. Even the painful experiences of world wars may have been passed on to the gene functions and sensations of subsequent generations.

Given the above account of research findings about how childhood and past generations affect pain symptoms in the here and now, a chronic pain sufferer may be inconsolable. However, these research findings don't mean that nothing can be done. Quite the contrary.

Although we bear the burden of previous generations, we also have many resourceful ways of coping with difficult situations and burdensome stages of life. The most important thing is to be aware that past issues have relevance and should not be swept under the carpet. Once you realise what the issue is, you can strive to break the cycle of generations. In spite of the past, you can live a good life as long as your own thoughts and actions focus on strengthening wellbeing rather than continuing to ruin it.

My own experience

I was brought up in the typical post-war culture in Finland with regard to touching and being touched. I have very few memories of being touched. We shook hands even among close relatives. I didn't even hug my own parents. Touch came into my life only in my youth, through sports. Among team members, high fives, pats on the back and hugs were part of happy moments and times of failure.

I haven't learned to manage my own pain through touch. Massage has never felt natural, not even when given by someone I love. Only now that I'm older and have read convincing studies about pain (I don't believe something until I see it) have I learned to seek out the healing touch and surrender to the analgesic effects of oxytocin.

Chronic pain affects a person's self-esteem and experience of self. In addition, it often affects couple relationships and sexual desire. These issues may be associated with shame and a sense of inferiority, which can be very difficult to face.

I wish I could talk about these topics more with my patients who suffer from pain; I'd want to hear their stories about being touched, tenderness and longing for human skin. Speaking about intimate matters isn't easy for either a patient or the doctor. It requires an adequate amount of time and trust for this aspect of a pain sufferer's life to surface. Both the treatment provider and the patient have to understand why these matters are important with respect to experiencing pain. They also need to realise that opening up about these matters can help to find ways of alleviating pain.

What you can do

- Anyone living with chronic pain knows that the symptoms come and go in waves. When pain symptoms are difficult, it's beneficial to invest particularly in pampering yourself. A bubble bath, massage, facial or visit to the health club may be the moment when a bad spell takes a turn for the better.
- If you're in a relationship where you think you aren't being touched enough, tell your partner. Say that your pain subsides when you're touched – if that is the case.
- Find a form of massage that suits you by trying different types. Traditional massage is good for some people while

effleurage, Shiatsu massage, Rosenberg therapy or hot stone massage may be good for others. Many options are available.

- Buy yourself several treatment sessions, or ask for them as a gift for a special occasion. You should have treatment once a week for at least five weeks. Affordable massage treatment may be offered by, among others, massage therapy schools.

- If you enjoy travel you can ask the hotel beforehand if they provide massage therapy services or they know a good local masseuse. You may be able to book the first appointment even for the same or following day of your flight.

- Massage must not be painful. If you experience pain or discomfort, tell your masseuse or masseur, as professionals can regulate the techniques and the amount of force applied according to the customer's wishes.

- If you're going for surgery or a painful procedure requiring anesthesia, while waiting you can try squeezing stress balls or stroking a stuffed animal. This really can help.

- To have sex, set aside a good amount of time and ensure a peaceful room, and try different types of sex or positions that don't cause pain. Sex can be more successful if you take a pain killer first. A Tantra yoga course can provide new enthusiasm for sexuality. You can even attend courses without a partner.

Chapter 5

Do what you enjoy

In life, you may encounter situations that make you revise your values and cause previously simple things to become challenges. A person disabled in a severe traffic accident may have to learn to walk again. Similarly, a chronic pain sufferer may also have to relearn the basics of everyday life. One of these basics is the ability to feel pleasure and enjoy oneself. Pain that has been a torment for a long time at worst destroys one's ability to enjoy life and feel happy. (For more about this see Chapter 6, Talk about your feelings.) Many people with chronic pain, just like people with depression, may therefore drift into making choices in their daily life that they know will worsen their wellbeing in the long term. Efforts to improve their life, in turn, are no longer rewarded as clearly as before because the person's capacity for enjoyment has diminished. What's more, it's hard to turn off the sense of feeling miserable. Even on a sunny day, the longing for the sofa in front of the TV is greater than the wish to go out for a walk. Your mind is like a little devil prodding you with a red-hot poker and whispering, 'It's useless to try, you'll only be disappointed and will fail – yet again.'

Along the way, the pain devil has perhaps made many things that once empowered you disappear from your life. For instance, physical activity, evenings at the theatre, travel, or shopping with friends may have ceased. Living with chronic pain may become restricted to carrying out small, essential routines, with few motivating bright spots.

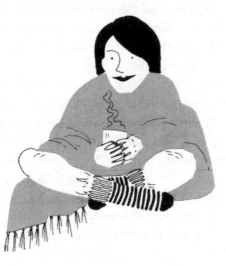

But I have good news for you: it's possible to regain the things you love. This doesn't require long periods of rehabilitation or courses on happiness, or drugs, or even much money. It's enough to follow a simple method that works for sure: you need only rediscover the things that bring you wellbeing and joy in life, revitalise your own daily life, and give this priority. One thing at a time.

Why pain sufferers should do what they enjoy

Major changes often start with minor actions. If your home is a bit too chilly, you wouldn't try to correct the situation by immediately starting a fundamental renovation, tearing down walls, replacing all the insulation, and rebuilding. The mere thought of such a difficult task is exhausting. The first thing you'd do is the most obvious: you'd close the window. Next, you'd put on your woolly socks and cardigan and begin to warm up nicely. At night you'd take a thicker blanket and would wake up in the morning after a good night's sleep. You'd rummage through your cupboards for your slightly worn but much loved sweater. At the same time you'd come across a box of old photographs, and pleasant memories of the past would come back to you as you looked through them. Perhaps you'd start to light the fire again – you'd forgotten how soothing the flames and quiet crackling of the fire could be.

While doing small things to dispel the cold, you'd find yourself experiencing brief moments of happiness.

This is exactly how you can also deal with your pain. It doesn't pay to lounge on the sofa and groan about the impossibility of a complete make-over. Instead, begin with the determination to add more activities, and things you enjoy doing, to your daily life, things you know will do you good. You may have to make some effort, just as you had to get up and go to your cupboards to dig around for a sweater. However, the effort will be rewarded.

Do something that brings you joy every day. Even if you can't manage to get out of bed one morning, you can still listen to good music, watch amusing videos for a couple of minutes, or phone a friend. The point is this: do some pleasant things for just a few minutes, if you can't manage to do any more. You can do more later, as long as you do something to make yourself feel better on a daily basis. Add another familiar activity you enjoy to your daily life every week. Or boldly try something new – but that, too, only a little at a time, at least initially.

Sew, tinker, decorate, arrange old photos, tend the garden – whatever inspires you. Do too little rather than too much, and rest in between. Stop in good time *before* you get sore, or, if you are in constant pain, before your pain gets worse. This is an important thing that requires a bit of practice. I'll try to explain it by means of an example – let that example be going to a flea market. (If that is not something you'd personally enjoy, bear with me – you can apply it to many other activities.) You know about how long you can manage to walk before pain arrives on the scene or gets worse. It could, for instance, be half an hour. When you get to the flea market, wander around for 20 minutes and then sit down for a moment to rest. In other words, sit down before you feel the worsening of your pain. After a brief rest, continue for another 10 to 15 minutes and then sit down again to rest. Don't stroll through the whole flea market, as you might have done in the past, but leave when you've been through half of it. Come back again, maybe the following week. Then, extend the time you're moving around, but by only a few minutes. Remember to stop and rest before your pain starts or gets worse. This is how you control your resilience and learn to anticipate pain. You unlearn detrimental thinking – 'I'll do this until it hurts and then I'll stop' – that reinforces pain through expectations. The goal is to teach your brain that going to the flea market is neither painful nor harmful.

Make time for yourself to do things that give you pleasure. Remember that it takes longer than before to do many familiar things, because of the pain, and this is just how it is. Act according to your present pace and don't bother about what others think. Whereas in the past you were able to weed your garden in a couple of hours, now it might take the whole day. Let your new goal be staying out in the garden long enough to get some weeds pulled up, even if only one small patch is clear. Glow with pleasure and praise yourself. For many individuals living with pain, an hour outdoors in the fresh air and a small job done are a fair achievement. A brief time outside being active is a much better option than doing nothing – which you may have been doing for quite some time, due to fear of pain. Tell yourself that gardening – or whatever equivalent you choose – isn't dangerous for you.

When you persistently add things that make you feel good to your everyday life, you'll soon see that happiness and joy begin to appear, at first peeping out shyly but gradually more courageously and lasting for longer. Feeling good pleases your body and your mind. You'll notice that your thinking is brighter and more flexible. As you feed positivity into your life, your interest in other people will begin to recover and your relationship with your partner will be refreshed. Without noticing it, you will start gliding towards a less painful state. It's important not to focus on determining whether you're happy now and how happy you are. You shouldn't strive for happiness; instead, you can let feeling good just come into your life with the help of small deeds.

Next I'll list additional changes you can include in your daily life and thus add to your pain management. A fair amount of research data has already accumulated about these measures.

Spoil yourself

I strongly believe in the importance of balance with regard to wellbeing and matters of health. A balanced life involves an appropriately varied assortment of things and activities, nothing too much or too little – whether food, drink, work, exercise, love, sex, hobbies, lounging... Healthy indulgence is a balancing factor that helps with pain management. Health-promoting indulgence is revitalising, whereas consoling oneself with, for instance, goodies and sweet 'treats' makes one sick. In my experience, the life of many chronic pain sufferers, myself included, involves too little self-nurturing and refreshing pampering and too much substitute activity with the intention of seeking comfort and offsetting the feeling of emptiness. A feature of healthy indulgence is seeing yourself in a positive and appreciative light. You're a good person and you take care of yourself, so you deserve pampering. So, give yourself a gift, something you know will enhance your wellbeing.

What research tells us

Water is one of the oldest treatments in medical history. This is supported by *The Kalevala*, my country's folklore-based national epic. Water has been used to treat people in spas for millennia, and the spa culture is still going strong in many countries. Several studies have been published internationally on water treatments in alleviating chronic pain. A visit to a spa is much more than pleasant relaxation and relief from the hustle and bustle of everyday life. Studies indicate that hydrotherapy (a type of physical therapy which uses water to create a therapeutic environment) and balneotherapy (treatments in mineral-rich waters and mud baths), especially if combined with in-water mobilisation movements or exercise, can relieve chronic pain, such as symptoms of fibromyalgia, chronic shoulder or back pain or rheumatic pain. The effects of water treatments have lasted at best for several months. In the UK, hydrotherapy is available on the NHS if an NHS physiotherapist recommends this after assessing you. Balneotherapy is generally not available in the UK as the mineral content of water is too weak; countries recommended for this treatment include Iceland, Bulgaria and Israel (the Dead Sea).

Warm water (32-33°C is recommended) improves blood circulation and relaxes the muscles. The pressure of water on the skin has a similar analgesic effect to touch, activating the nerve endings under the skin; the messages despatched from these nerve endings prevent the transmission of pain signals to the brain (more detail on this in Chapter 4). As a result of both hydrotherapy and balneotherapy, the brain is stimulated to secrete endorphins and our own pain regulation system begins to wake up again. Related indicators in the blood start to improve too. Recent research data show improvement in blood values for inflammation (these go down), cortisol levels and levels of problematic fats in the blood, as well as an increase in body-repairing growth factors in the bloodstream. In hydrotherapy, exercising in water is an essential aspect of the analgesic effect (more about this in Chapter 8). In addition, the beautiful and often peaceful atmosphere of a therapeutic swimming pool or spa calms the mind and body, at best in the same way as meditation. Whether the minerals in the water really contribute to pain tolerance is still not known reliably.

What you can do – How to benefit most from indulging yourself

- Ask your GP to refer you for possible hydrotherapy. As I have said, hydrotherapy sessions are available on the NHS if you meet the relevant criteria. Arthritis Research UK published an information booklet in 2016, *What is Hydrotherapy?* It can be accessed via www.arthritisresearchuk.org/arthritis-information/therapies/hydrotherapy/what-is-hydrotherapy.aspx. In the UK hydrotherapy is most used for rheumatoid and/or inflammatory arthritis and other rheumatic conditions. A qualified physiotherapist will be registered with the Health Professionals Council (HPC), and it's recommended that you see someone who is a member of the Chartered Society of Physiotherapists (CSP) and who is accredited by the Aquatic Therapy Association of Chartered Physiotherapists (ATACP).
- In Britain, there are many private health centres that offer water treatments. If your loved ones are planning to get you a birthday present, suggest that you'd like a gift voucher to such a centre.
- Also, when selecting a holiday destination abroad, you can choose a country with a long tradition of hydrotherapy and other spa treatments. These include, among others, Hungary and Estonia.
- However, there isn't always money or time for indulgence in a private health centre. Public swimming pools may have whirlpools and hydromassage showers that can be very helpful.
- A bath at home is also an excellent way to relax the body and mind.

Visualise your 'soul's landscape'

Pain can also be alleviated by visualisation exercises. As I've mentioned earlier in this book, by looking at real-time images of their own brain activity on the computer screen during functional magnetic resonance imaging, a person can learn to train the functioning of their brain and, at the same time, to relieve pain by means of visualisation exercises. The functioning and structure of the brain can be altered by visualisation exercises and various sensory illusions, which trick the brain. Pain management for phantom-limb pain and other types of chronic limb pain utilises, for instance, mirror therapy: the patient watches in a mirror the reflection of their healthy limb in the place of their painful limb hidden behind the mirror, and, using this vision image, teaches their brain to reduce its experience of pain. Even though we know what we see and experience aren't real, the brain processes these observations as though they were.

One of the easiest visualisation exercises is what I call 'visualising the soul's landscape'. This doesn't require either money or leaving home. Just sit or lie still, close your eyes, and concentrate on your favourite place – a place where both body and soul are at rest. In the soul's landscape you're in a safe place, protected from pain.

What research tells us

Danish researchers recently conducted a study that tested visualising the soul's landscape (the place where participants felt safe and pain-free) in conjunction with a fairly major procedure – cardiac ablation to treat severe heart arrhythmia, in which, under local anaesthetic, a catheter is guided to the heart via the femoral vein. The procedure is quite challenging and is often experienced as being painful and even frightening.

Before and during the procedure, patients were asked to transfer their thoughts to a favourite place where they felt safe.

Many thought of their summer cottage or a lovely sandy beach in the sun. A good many went to the forest – in their imagination, that is. Research has shown the forest/woodland to be a refreshing and calming place. (By the way, some studies published in recent years have found that chronic pain, symptoms of depression, and stress can in fact be alleviated by walking in the forest/among trees.)

But back to the procedure where patients were asked to sense the scents and sounds of their favourite place and to focus on its tranquil ambience. The wonderful warmth of the sand, the gentle touch of a soft breeze, the fresh smell of the forest. It was a pleasure to be in this favourite place, free of cares and troubles. This sort of simple visualisation exercise reduced the experience of pain and the need for analgesics both during the procedure and after it. By visualising their 'soul's landscape', patients felt that they were able to manage their pain better.

This method can be used when you're going for a procedure that you know will be unpleasant or painful. You can also try it at home when you feel your own pain is worsening or if anxiety and worry squeeze your chest. Look at a picture of your favourite place first, then close your eyes for a moment and be transported there in your mind.

What you can do – How to benefit from visualisation techniques

- You can imagine that your chronic pain has some other form. It might be a loud sound or an annoyingly bright lamp. In your mind, learn how to dim the light with the switch or make the sound quieter with the control knob. You can also imagine that your brain begins pumping large amounts of morphine into your bloodstream and that this eases the pain.
- Focus your thoughts on some other part of your body that

isn't painful. Imagine that that place starts to feel warm. Or, in your mind slowly transfer your back pain to a place where it's easier to manage – say, to your hand.

- An experienced physiotherapist who understands the psychophysiology of chronic pain comprehensively can guide you in these exercises.
- More information about visualisation exercises can be found on the internet, for example at Pain Support UK: https://painsupport.co.uk/pain-relief/visualisation/

Maintain social relationships

Friendship is 'a single soul dwelling in two bodies', as Aristotle once beautifully put it. Although chronic pain eats at strength and tries to set limits on how we live, friendship should still be cherished. No matter how they're measured, social support and a sense of community are among the most important sources of health, wellbeing and happiness. Their beneficial effect on health is roughly the same as that of not smoking – and three times more important than ideal weight, as a systematic review and meta-analysis involving over 300,000 people indicated. Thus, by maintaining social relationships you can achieve as good or even better health than by avoiding smoking or losing weight. The perfect win–win situation: friendship and wellbeing!

Everyone, but especially a person with chronic pain, wants and deserves approval and appreciation, and the experience of being listened to and understood without judgement, disparagement or recrimination. Chronic pain and the associated fatigue, however, inevitably pose challenges for social interaction. Physical pain also sensitises a person to social pain. It may be a consequence of the way the brain, already over-sensitive due to pain, interprets what the environment says, and leaves unsaid, in an overly negative way.

Identify your own sensitivity to interpreting other people's actions and behaviour and think about how to turn it into a strength. Learn to read people's non-verbal communication, especially the way they look at you. The eyes are the mirror of our feelings. How one person looks at another can convey many beautiful and gentle things that aren't said aloud. There are many people in the world who have no need or wish to belittle or invalidate you and your symptoms. It pays to give new people the chance to be kind and understanding – despite previous negative experiences. Trust that you are interesting and can fit in just as well as others. Most of all, you shouldn't be afraid that your established lifestyle will be derailed as your social life expands. The train of life stays on the rails, but good company makes the trip much more pleasant.

What research tells us

At its worst, chronic pain causes isolation and leads to loneliness, but things may also play out differently: loneliness may maintain or worsen the body's inflammatory reactions which, in turn, may underlie pain. Loneliness and chronic pain have astonishingly similar effects on the body. Both over-sensitise the central nervous system to detect potential threats coming from the environment. Pain is perceived as a danger signal even if there is no longer any real danger. The threat of loneliness, on the other hand, is associated with other people, their attitudes and critical ways of expressing themselves.

One isn't necessarily aware of this oversensitisation of the nervous system, but it can be observed, for example, in sleep measurements: the sleep of a person who lives alone is often more fitful because the sleeper is subconsciously on guard in case of an emergency and therefore sleeps lightly, awakened by every noise. Broken sleep in turn worsens pain (more about this topic in Chapter 2, Value your sleep).

Few health problems cause as much social isolation as chronic pain. As a physician, I have often sensed a pain patient's

loneliness even if he or she hasn't brought it up. It is common –
and very human and understandable – that a pain patient begins
to protect himself or herself from the mental pain experienced
when symptoms are disparaged and invalidated. The individual
may become cynical and build a protective shell that has a
negative charge. The protective shell works for a while and
deflects comments that are interpreted as negative. But in the
end, the only way to prevent the protective shell from collapsing
is to avoid encountering others.

Positive support from other pain sufferers can dispel the fears
of a person with chronic pain. It emboldens, encourages and
helps a person who stumbles to get back on their feet. Another
person who has had similar experiences can offer empathy and
understanding, and doesn't judge or accuse. Support from other
pain sufferers helps the person succeed in getting a grip on pain
and life. A support group provides a place to experience a sense
of belonging with people who understand the life of a person
with chronic pain. Pain need not be explained or defended in the
group; instead, one can 'come out of the closet' with regard to
pain – and no one will turn their back.

Empowerment through another person occurs best by means
of face-to-face encounters, looking the other person in the eye.
Sometimes, however, it's necessary to resort to other means.
Fortunately, there are groups on the internet and via social media
where a chronic pain sufferer can seek peer support. In closed
groups on Facebook, there are hundreds if not thousands of
people, so the amount of potential support is huge. The group can
become a new family-like community to a person with pain. The
few studies that have reported on the effect of social media on
the life of a person with chronic pain have shown that there is a
need for these groups. In the studies, respondents have mainly
felt that they have received additional mental and social wellbeing
through the groups. At best, self-efficacy and the feeling of being
able to cope increase with the positive support of peers.

On the other hand, all forms of social media are also known

to have another side. More about the negatively oriented sensitivity of the brain is found in Chapter 3, Discover the importance of positive thinking. According to research, social media provides a place where people are more likely to unburden themselves of their unhappiness than to share their experiences of success. It's important for individuals to be able to speak about their emotions, including negative ones. This is exactly why peer support groups on the internet are experienced as particularly necessary. However, negativity may be over-emphasised in these online groups so the impression that emerges is not representative of the whole picture of living with pain. Discussion on the internet can inadvertently reinforce the image of hopelessness and the endless cycle of injustice encountered by pain patients in relation to healthy people, healthcare professionals or the authorities. Tips on care shared in the group can trigger contradictory feelings, as they may differ widely from conventional care practices.

Being in constant contact with an online group can also stealthily increase a person's observation of his/her own pain symptoms. According to brain research, increased focus on symptoms increases the electrical activation of pain sensing areas in the brain and thus maintains pain. A similar, somewhat surprising effect has been found for keeping a pain diary. A Canadian study has shown that people with back pain who kept a pain diary recovered significantly less well than those who weren't asked to record their daily symptoms. The study concluded by recommending, with good reason, that keeping pain diaries should be avoided. Online group updates can function in the same way as a sort of diary. In addition, it is known that, as a feeling, pain may be 'catching': listening to and watching another person's suffering activates largely the same areas of the brain as when the pain is experienced by oneself. At its worst, an online group that rehashes negative emotions and experiences can maintain the pain symptoms of its members and strengthen the feeling of being ill. At its best, however, in many ways the group empowers and reinforces the individual's own ways of coping with pain.

The positive effects of group activities can be increased by discussing, with the other group members, the reliability of shared information and by encouraging others to share experiences of successful pain management and coping. Group administrators can act as initiators and coordinators in this. One way to endorse empowerment is to use art and culture, the health-promoting effects of which are supported by good practical experience and research findings. The sharing of inspiring photos, pieces of music, films, writing, poems, etc. in groups has been found to have positive effects. (For more about this see Chapter 17, Be creative.)

What you can do – How to make the most of relationships

- National and local pain patient associations organise peer support activities. Contact details can be found online, e.g., https://painuk.org/
- Not everyone thrives in a group, but peer support can also be obtained by phone and on the internet, or by asking the support person to pay a visit to one's home. Some of the pain associations have a closed Facebook group that can be joined by sending a request to the group's administrators. You can also meet new people through hobbies. Particularly suitable for pain patients are singing, dancing, music, car tuning and handicrafts. The internet has abundant information about dance or craft clubs or choirs, e.g. www.choirs.org.uk/home.htm.
- Friendships should be maintained and cared for in the same way as a beautiful garden so they can flourish and bring joy and energy. Don't forget to tell your loved ones what their friendship means to you and how it helps you to cope despite your pain.

Play

You're home on Saturday night. Pain has tormented you badly and you haven't been able to do much more than lie about. Once again, the medications you've taken haven't warded off the pain and you're wondering what to do. Normally, you might stay on the sofa watching TV because you haven't got the strength to do anything else, but you find you can't concentrate on any of the programmes because you can't take your mind off the pain. You wonder whether you should take yet another painkiller – maybe this time it would ease the pain and you wouldn't feel so aggravated?

What if you were to try playing something? You could dig out an old pack of playing cards or turn on your computer and click on a game of patience or sudoku. With good music playing in the background, you might soon notice that it's fun to play. You might find yourself singing along with the songs and get so wrapped up in the game that your pain would be forgotten for a while.

If I could secretly use functional MRI to get an image of your cerebral cortex, I would be able to show you how beautifully the electric scramble in areas that sense pain calms down in this scenario. That's why the pain eases up. By playing board games or video games or computer games, piecing together jigsaw puzzles, or solving crossword puzzles, your thoughts concentrate on meaningful activity where you need to use your wits. Your attention is focused away from pain, and your pain is consequently relieved. The need for painkillers is probably lessened. You develop as you play: determination, perseverance and optimism begin to increase and you experience modest feelings of success – which may otherwise be scarce in your life.

It isn't always this easy to draw attention away from pain, and the strength of the pain may not necessarily explain whether or not this is successful. As is well known, everybody is different: some people pay more attention to pain than others, making pain harder 'to turn off'; whereas others become absorbed in interesting challenges despite distractions such as pain.

What research tells us

Playing games/doing puzzles has made it possible to carry out difficult and painful procedures, such as changing a burn patient's dressings, with much less pain and smaller doses of painkillers. In recent years, pain rehabilitation has also begun to take advantage of gaming and moving around in the virtual world. In the virtual world, a person experiencing pain can practise things that he otherwise wouldn't believe he could do because of fear that the pain or its underlying cause might worsen. The virtual world makes it possible to bypass the overprotection originating in the brain. Body movement can be improved, and ability and the feeling of coping can be increased, by cheating the brain: the game or the virtual world feeds the player's 'observations' that deviate from reality. Without realising it, people use their body more bravely and then happily find that the movement didn't worsen the pain after all.

Many great virtual methods have been developed and are used in pain rehabilitation. While walking on a treadmill, a pain patient can simultaneously gaze at a magnificent sandy beach or metropolis watching a screen in from of him/her. Or s/he can create a virtual figure, an avatar, which is then used to move about in a simulated world full of pleasant, interesting details. A new limb, guided by movement measured from the stump, has been created virtually for amputees. As s/he looks at the movement of his/her virtual limb with virtual reality glasses, the amputee has felt the movement and the brain has observed that the movement doesn't produce pain. Phantom-limb pain has been alleviated through exercises of this type.

In a gaming application meant for people with back pain, a small sensor is taped to the skin of the back, and on the computer a video game is played that allows the back pain sufferer, for example, to ski downhill, dance and do yoga exercises virtually. The sensor takes the necessary measurements and guides the back to make the right movements. Such games, which are suitable for use at home, will surely become more common in the near future.

What you can do – How you can benefit from play

- The computer is, once again, an inexhaustible source of information. If you want to learn a new card game, instructions can be found online, for instance at www. pagat.com. Challenge your friends, for example, to a game of online backgammon, or accept the challenge to play against a stranger (you can use a pseudonym to play).
- Organise an evening of playing board games at your home or check out if there are any game nights in your locality. More information is available on the website of The Royal Society of Gamers www.royalsocietyofgamers. com. The website also has instructions for setting up your own game club.
- If you aren't already familiar with video games, ask a clever relative or friend to guide you through the options. Most are quite easy to play, and you are sure to find an appropriate level. Be brave and give it a try!
- Playing can be combined with enjoyable competition and movement. Starting and maintaining movement at home by means of video gaming can be easier than going out for a walk.

Relax

Stress comes on automatically, without any particularly strong stimulus, but relaxing doesn't occur automatically; it requires conscious effort. It's a skill that needs to be learned and repeated enough to become automatic – just like learning to ride a bike. You can develop your skills – to put it more technically, you can 'condition yourself' – so much that when you simply tell yourself 'relax', you're be able to do so completely, right away. This does, however, require quite a lot of practice.

In order to manage pain, numerous relaxation exercises have been developed that aim to balance the functioning of the two parts of the involuntary, or 'autonomic', nervous system: to curb the overactivity of the sympathetic (accelerating) nervous system, and strengthen the functioning of the parasympathetic (calming) nervous system. The physiological effects can be measured immediately: the pulse stabilises, blood pressure drops, breathing deepens, muscle oxygenation improves and muscles relax. However, most important with regard to pain management are the effects of relaxation on stress tolerance, emotional control and the ability to concentrate.

It's quite easy to do relaxation training; it doesn't require much money, and the risks are minimal. A person with chronic pain should make relaxation exercises a way of life, doing them repeatedly, preferably on a daily basis. Their effect can be enhanced by combining them with other means of pain management, such as thinking about positive things, humour or social get-togethers.

What research tells us

The most research-based evidence has accumulated for the treatment of migraine. The effect of relaxation exercises on migraine has been on a par with pharmacotherapy (medication) – that is, the frequency of headache attacks and the intensity of pain decrease on average by 30 to 50 per cent. That's a pretty good result.

Pharmacotherapy is, of course, much quicker: just take a pill and swallow it. Learning and carrying out relaxation exercises require commitment and take time – albeit only 10–20 minutes a day, or a few times a week. I often hear my patients say that they wouldn't want to take any medications even though these might be helpful. If this sort of medication-free treatment mode has the same result as taking drugs, and certainly has fewer adverse effects, it's worth trying.

Despite extensive use, so far there isn't a great deal of reliable scientific evidence on the effects – especially the longer-term effectiveness – of relaxation exercises and therapies in other chronic pain conditions. I think their full potential hasn't yet been discovered because people may not necessarily be able to relax if they have a lot of pain-related worries and fears. Worries should therefore be dispelled before relaxation is possible.

Relaxation exercises, however, seem to be an excellent additional help for the ordinary companions of pain – insomnia, anxiety and a depressed state of mind. Relaxation taking place through the 'biofeedback method' is beneficial for many people with fibromyalgia and painful temporomandibular disorders, at least in the short term. The method is learned by using a separate electronic device to control and reduce muscle tension.

Convincing scientific evidence of any benefits from relaxation based on deep breathing techniques and diaphragmatic exercises has not yet been produced.

What you can do – How you can learn to relax

- Learn to recognise the effects of muscle tension and stress in your body. This is beneficial in pain management: you can better recognise the worsening of your pain and act in time.
- So-called 'applied relaxation', which includes five different methods, is widely used in Finland where I work. Progressive muscle relaxation is one of these. It involves tightening each muscle group, such as the thigh muscles,

one by one for five seconds and then relaxing for 30 seconds. This relaxation can be implemented anywhere, at any time. (See www.nhsinform.scot/healthy-living/preventing-falls/fear-and-anxiety-about-falling/relaxation-techniques)

- Physiotherapists are able to advise and guide you with regard to different relaxation techniques. You can ask them about biofeedback therapy. Relaxation exercises can be learned alone at home with the help of a CD or the internet (there are relevant videos on YouTube), or in a group. You can also ask your local health centre/GP practice or association for pain patients about relaxation groups. There are many pain management courses which teach relaxation. (See www.nhs.uk/live-well/healthy-body/10-ways-to-ease-pain/)
- If one particular relaxation technique doesn't suit you, try another. Don't give up even if your efforts aren't rewarded in the form of pain relief right away. It takes on average 60 days to learn a new thing and benefit from it.

My own experience

Could my back pain be malignant after all? Might I have a stroke at some time because of these terrible migraines? Will I need hip replacement surgery in the coming years? Is this what my life is going to be – struggling with pain? Will I lose my ability to work?

Such thoughts go through the mind of everyone with chronic pain, myself included. I started to benefit from relaxation exercises only when my fears eased up. It took quite a long time. Needless to say, my worries and distress have not completely gone, but I'm less anxious about my pain than I used to be. It was crucial to understand and accept that some of my pain symptoms were maintained by my central nervous system. 'Brain pain' is what I call this kind of pain. It cannot be surgically removed nor is it completely curable by any other method. However, my pain isn't a sign of danger or damage and it won't destroy me. In fact, I've begun to think that some of my pain symptoms are an irritating complaint in the same sort of way as tinnitus (ringing in the ears) – one shouldn't pay them any mind. I tell myself that what my basic pain is trying to communicate is of no importance to me. I can consciously influence that aspect of my pain very well by relaxing.

I can't really say I'm very good at relaxation, nor can I manage to do the exercises for very long or earnestly. I learn new, quicker means all the time. The most suitable for me is a short relaxation exercise either in the bath or just before falling asleep. At an applied relaxation course, I learned a quick (roughly two-minute) relaxation method that at times I try to do at my desk. It's not that easy and I don't always have the stamina to go through my whole body. It's easier to do a few minutes of mindfulness breathing exercises. I can't get into relaxation mood without first giving myself permission to relax. I know this sounds funny, but I have to engage in dialogue with myself. I say that I have the right to relax, that I don't have to achieve all the time. Things will be dealt with later. Only then can I do the relaxation exercise.

Relaxation in water is particularly successful. The aching body longs for warm water now and then. For me, a bath in my own tub is a little everyday luxury that produces both physical pain relief and mental wellbeing. When travelling, I choose a hotel room with a bathtub, if one is available. After a long day at a congress, it's wonderful to slip into a warm bubble bath. I've also begun to be an active user of the 'soul's landscape' training, both in my own pain management and in my work with patients. When my body is on fire or the dentist injects an anaesthetic, or I just want to calm my mind, I transfer my thoughts to the warm sandy beaches of the South or to my little cottage where I can watch the sunset. I feel better instantly. Migraine is the only pain for which I find visualisation exercises are ineffective.

Chapter 5

I give my patients a cortisone injection occasionally; so that the shot hurts as little as possible, I ask them beforehand to think about their favourite place. I do likewise before and during acupuncture treatments. I've found that this works, and in addition, the acupuncture is probably more effective when combined with a visualisation exercise. The power of the mind is verifiably awesome!

Finally, at the end of this long chapter, here are my own experiences of friendship. It is very difficult to maintain social relationships when pain gnaws away and consumes one's strength and one's thoughts no longer hold together in the evening, at the end of the working day. Going for a walk with a friend can't be agreed in advance because I never know whether it will be possible to walk very far in the evening. I wouldn't want to explain why walking is so difficult or why I haven't made an appointment for physiotherapy. I'm no longer eager to arrange dinner parties because the mere idea of cleaning the house thoroughly and putting together a complicated menu is exhausting (as if there were no other options!). I can't drink alcohol anymore because of migraine, and that also seems to be a social limitation. However, I'm sustained by the understanding that these limitations exist mainly in my head. Pain chips away at self-esteem and makes things look black and white. It's been surprising to see how easily the feeling of inferiority creeps into my mind and how withdrawal from social events becomes increasingly natural. From time to time, the pain devil can isolate even someone as naturally social as myself.

Yet a phone call from a friend or an invitation to a party at a friend's home always delights. After meeting friends, I swear to myself that I'll start to be more active again because I always get more strength from these encounters. The longing for social interaction is fortunately so strong that I won't give in to pain with respect to that, either. And secretly I hope that my friends don't give up and realise what a tremendous resource they are in my life even though I can't always express it verbally.

Chapter 6

Talk about your feelings

Speaking about their emotions is one of the most important and effective ways for people with chronic pain to head off the worsening of pain and to prevent everyday life from becoming a torment. Speaking about one's emotions can be learned. It isn't even that hard. It's harder to learn to recognise one's own feelings, to face them for what they are as they come, and to allow oneself to have feelings at all.

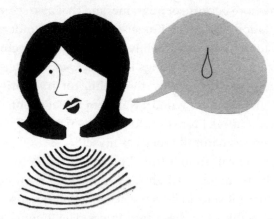

The colour grey isn't merely grey; there are countless different shades. The big dark cloud over our head, which is so familiar to many people with chronic pain, has many shades, many distinct emotional states, once one has learned to see them.

Disappointment lies within the cloud. Sorrow, shame, and anger also live there. They are all a part of your pain.

As you continue to observe your feelings, you'll find that many positive emotions are there as well, emotions that have been trampled by pain, anger and disappointment. There, stamina raises its head, as do self-worth, gratitude and passion, as well as cheerfulness and courage. They are all emotion-based tools for pain management, which should be harnessed for use.

Why people suffering from pain should talk about their feelings

Emotions have great power to maintain health. They also make people ill. Although it's empowering to cultivate positivity (there is more about this in Chapter 3, Discover the importance of positive thinking), for the sake of health and pain management it's important to leave room for negative emotions as well. If you suppress emotions, they desperately seek a way out and finally break through as physical symptoms. Many chronic pain sufferers suppress their own emotions, whether out of embarrassment or a sense of guilt, or to protect themselves or others from unpleasant feelings.

For you to be able to cope with your pain better, you must be able to be yourself, with all of your own thoughts and feelings. You should not have to hide your own situation in order to make yourself inconspicuous or acceptable. You shouldn't give priority to the feelings of others, and you don't always have to do everything in your power to keep others from being disappointed. You don't have to care so much about what others think, and you don't have to try to please in order to gain approval. You aren't responsible for the feelings of anyone except yourself. When emotions are allowed to come out in their true form, they may for a moment be difficult to express and stretch the limits of your comfort zone so that you feel something like a temporary increase in pain. However, they gradually find their own form and place – and the pain eases up. The cloud begins to disperse.

What research tells us

When the mood of healthy subjects has been lightened in a test laboratory – for example, by telling amusing stories – their pain threshold has risen quickly and the pain caused during the experiment has started to feel more tolerable. At the same time, the nerve activity in the brain cortex areas relating to pain has slowed down. Depressing the mood by berating or intimidating participants, or playing melancholic music, in turn, has been shown to cause the opposite reaction: the brain is activated to sense pain more sharply and the experience of pain is intensified.

The situation for those with fibromyalgia seems to be different: lightening the mood doesn't necessarily affect their pain threshold. For many, it's the same whether the mood is happy or sad, the pain is still experienced as strongly. In studies, chronic pain sufferers have been found to have more difficulties in handling and expressing feelings than people without pain. They may avoid dealing with emotions, or they may suppress them. The emotions experienced are primarily more negative, and perhaps for that reason feelings are expressed less often (this is discussed more in Chapter 5, Do what you enjoy).

The longer pain lasts, the more strongly emotions inevitably enter into the picture. The more vague the pain is, with no clear cause found, the more uncertainty it generates. Uncertainty, in turn, causes stress, frustration, apprehension and anxiety, while prolonged pain increases depression as well as feelings of anger and even sorrow.

Stress

The feeling of **stress** is familiar to all of us. Stress can be a good thing when it is short in duration, as it makes us act, achieve goals and stick to deadlines. Thanks to good stress, we are energetic and productive. Stress may, however, become burdensome and depressing if the factor causing it is prolonged, repeated or excessively intense.

Everyone reacts to stress differently. Studies have shown that it can trigger or strengthen various pain states, such as headaches, facial pain, back pain, abdominal cramps and fibromyalgia. According to current understanding, stress increases pain by sensitising and weakening the functioning of downward-oriented pain braking systems (the so-called 'descending pain inhibitory system' from the brain to the spinal cord). Stress also increases the activity of the sympathetic nervous system and strengthens fears, which in turn worsen the pain experience.

Anxiety

Many people with chronic pain have **fears** that are not easy to discuss: concern that pain will worsen and worries about drug addiction; fear that their spouse will wilt: 'Soon s/he won't be able to listen any more; s/he'll look for someone young and healthy.' There may also be the fear of losing their job and their ability to work. Or fear of what staying with the job might do to pain. In addition, there are often financial concerns.

In 2013, American researchers published a large-scale meta-study (where all relevant previous research is reviewed) encompassing almost 10,000 people examined for pain symptoms. This study, one of the biggest published on the subject, confirmed the long-held concept that the fears linked to pain are associated with inability to function. The connection is strong: the more fears the person has, the more disabling the pain is considered to be and the worse the functioning is. This doesn't seem to be affected by age, gender, the location of pain in the body, the strength of pain or by how long pain has lasted. Fear in itself may be more discouraging than the tissue damage possibly underlying the pain.

Depression

Another emotion that easily discourages the chronic pain sufferer is **depression**. A depressed mood is a very common companion of pain. Pain causes various emotions, including depression. Depression, in turn, can manifest itself as unspecific pain symptoms. Not all people suffering from chronic pain feel depressed, and not all of those who are depressed suffer from more pain symptoms than usual. It is very common, however, for the two to occur simultaneously.

Symptoms of depression clearly increase the risk of back pain. The risk among people with severe depression is about 2.5 times that of people with mild depression. Even slight depression significantly increases the risk that back pain will surface. More than half of the patients at pain clinics – in some studies as many as 80 per cent – can be diagnosed as having clinical depression. One out of four pain sufferers who seek help at primary health care level (from their GP/family doctor) have symptoms of depression. Depression, however, may remain unnoticed because most pain sufferers seek help only for their physical complaint. Or, within the framework of the short time of the appointment, attention is focused on the physical complaint and there isn't the time, or the knowledge, or sometimes the courage, to ask about the sufferer's mental state. The pain symptom may mask depression, which thus remains unrecognised, without diagnosis or treatment.

Pain and depression together – and especially if accompanied by poor sleep – prolong sick leaves, make people more vulnerable to permanent disability, and ruin quality of life. That's why both need to be treated regardless of which is the cause and which is the consequence. If only pain is treated, without simultaneously treating depression, the pain usually doesn't improve. Or if the focus is on treating depression and pain is not managed, the person's spirits aren't necessarily raised.

Anger

Expressing emotions is beneficial. However, one should be careful with **anger**. Anger is a feeling that easily takes over. There's nothing wrong with feeling angry, but when it comes to expressing it, it may quickly get out of hand. There are people who experience intense feelings of anger and express them forcefully, venting them on their surroundings, their loved ones or, for instance, on the internet. Studies show that people suffering from anger management problems tend to feel stronger pain and their mood is more negative. Pain reinforces anger and anger strengthens pain.

A pain sufferer's uncontrolled eruption of anger and frustration activates the defence mechanisms of loved ones, care givers or the employer, thus further increasing their rebuffs. When angry, a person suffering from pain may become unfriendly, difficult or even intolerable in the eyes of others. On the other hand, the repression of anger by all means doesn't make one feel any better. One should learn constructive ways to control and express anger. There are some tips at the end of this chapter, under the heading 'What you can do – How to manage your emotions'.

Many people who struggle with chronic pain experience losses in their life: the physical being seems to decay, strength decreases, joy and enthusiasm disappear, friendships fade; it's no longer possible to continue the interests that used be so enjoyable. Work becomes harder, and the ability to withstand stress all but disappears. These are difficult issues, major changes in life, and their significance should not be underestimated.

Sorrow

Our natural reaction in the face of loss is to grieve. **Sorrow** is an emotion that should be acknowledged and allowed to accompany us in life for a while. Sorrow helps us to adapt; by grieving, we can gradually begin to feel better and new hope arises through sorrow. Hope grows when one encounters and accepts the reality of one's life at that particular moment. However, sorrow isn't the same as worrying. Worrying keeps grinding away at the same issues and the same pain, maintaining anxiety and pain.

Some time ago I read a study where three out of four chronic pain sufferers felt that they were a burden to their loved ones or family members. It must be an upsetting and contradictory feeling, because without the help of loved ones it may be difficult or impossible to survive. The feeling of being a burden increases the pain and depression, and can even lead to self-destructive thoughts. If you feel this way, think about why it is you do so and what you can do to change the feeling. It's possible to learn to rely on others less and to find within yourself the capable and skilled person you used to be. You should also ask your loved ones about their feelings and expectations, and listen to them. They may well have ideas about how existing roles can be changed. It's almost certain that they would prefer to increase your feelings of coping and capability through their actions instead of unintentionally increasing your feeling of being a burden.

My own experience

As a young doctor, many times when treating pain sufferers I found myself wondering why the emotions linked with pain weren't discussed. Patients with awkward and long-term pain often only reported experiencing pain. Although their ability to work had gone and life was limited to within four walls, with no cure or even alleviating treatment available, pain was what people spoke about together with amazement that neither cause nor treatment could be found for the pain. There was no mention of frustration, sorrow, disappointments, feelings of anger towards the pain, or of fears. Only talk of physical pain.

Now as a more experienced doctor, through pain research and my own experiences with pain, I've realised why this is the case. I understand that it's easier for many to handle pain through the idea of tissue damage. Opening the door to emotions may seem like opening a Pandora's box, and that's why it may seem better to keep the mind separate from the body. Many physicians and other healthcare professionals may also think this way – that it's better not to ask about emotions since no treatment is available. Maybe the unpleasant feelings will go away by themselves if they're not brought up. The care-giver perhaps can't tolerate the feeling of helplessness that the emotions of the pain patient awaken in him/her.

Many pain patients learn to keep quiet about their affairs and feelings for fear of having them belittled and invalidated. Pain sensitises people's attitudes and even makes them cynical. People use cynicism and sarcasm for protection, but the effects on themselves and on the environment are detrimental. When the amount of joy is reduced, negativity becomes the normal state without this being noticed.

Joy is not unknown to chronic pain sufferers. When encountered, it gets a warm reception and is appreciated and cherished. Many things bring joy: the attentiveness and smiles of other people, the empathy and understanding of care-givers, a small word of thanks from a supervisor or fellow worker. Positive emotions awaken from their slumber in no time; the eyes brighten and it's again easier to cope with the pain.

I've learned the hard way that the emotions raging within readily distort reality. Feelings can prevent us from hearing and understanding what that the doctor or other healthcare professional says. The emotional state selects information that suits it. A depressed person will only hear the doctor say 'The pain won't get better', even though the sentence continues '... but it can be managed and you can live a good life with it.' After consultation with an orthopaedic surgeon, the fearful patient remembers only the words '... we'll consider surgery', even though the doctor has said, 'First we'll try other approaches and only then we'll consider surgery.' If feelings related to pain are churning in the mind, it's advisable to take a support person with you to the doctor's office or other treatments, as this person will hear what's said and make observations without the interference of pain-generated emotional storms. (More about my own sorrow associated with pain can be found in the introductory chapter, My own story.)

What you can do – How to manage your emotions

- Emotions come and go, but they don't define you as a person. If you feel sorrow, that doesn't make you a sad person. If you have symptoms of depression, it doesn't mean that you are a depressed person.
- Learn to separate facts from your feelings. Chronic pain is a fact of life. The other related experiences are mainly emotions.
- Denying rather than accepting chronic pain may lead to despair, anxiety and running from one doctor to the next in the hope of finding a quick fix. It would help you better to seek a doctor or other professional who understands chronic pain, gives you enough time and takes you and your pain into account as a whole.
- Talk about your emotions related to pain. If you're depressed or have fears going round in your head, tell your loved ones and your healthcare professional. As far as depression is concerned, it's not enough only to recognise it. Depression must also be treated.
- The feeling of inferiority associated with chronic pain may cause withdrawal from others and isolation. Be compassionate and merciful to yourself. When you appreciate yourself, you will want to do your best to manage your pain. Seek the company of people who support you in your goals.
- Because we are all human, the fears and attitudes of healthcare professionals affect their work, too. If your

doctor only suggests rest and sick leave as treatment for chronic pain, don't settle for that. Insist on discussing other options as well and/or request a second opinion.

- Vent frustration, annoyance and anger calmly by talking, writing, exercising, dancing, cleaning, splitting firewood, or even shouting in the quiet of the countryside. They all are better ways than ranting and raving.
- Identify the sources of your anger before it takes over and think about how you'll act next time rage appears on the scene. Learn to take time-out by counting to 10, looking out of the window or going for a walk. It often pays to sleep on the matter before sending a letter or a message where you let out your internal anger.
- It's worth learning to recognise and talk about emotions. This is difficult alone, but it isn't impossible. Take advantage of professional know-how for this.
- A number of studies have shown that many forms of counselling are helpful in managing pain. These include, among others, cognitive behaviour therapy (CBT) that explores, identifies and modifies harmful thinking, behaviour and emotions, and acceptance and commitment therapy. Ask your doctor about available therapies or read more about the subject on the internet – for instance, here: www.apa.org/helpcenter/pain-management.aspx.

Chapter 7

Eat wisely

A physician in Ancient Greece called Hippocrates was a wise man. His views revolutionised the medical science of his day and he is, with reason, considered to be the 'father of Western medicine'. He was among the first to have a sceptical view of what were then thought to be the reasons for diseases. He understood that they didn't stem from the gods' anger and punishment, but had quite natural causes. Nature, according to him, could also heal diseases, and the doctor needed only actively to assist nature.

Hippocrates cleverly concluded that treatment for a disease shouldn't harm the patient, an idea that was not self-evident at a time of bloodletting, poisonous concoctions and skull drilling! He showed particular insight when he stated that disease couldn't be understood unless the patient was seen holistically, as a whole person. He emphasised the importance of balance as the basis of health. Exercise, nutrition, water treatments and sunbathing were therefore integral elements of his treatment regimens. Hippocrates learned, and taught his colleagues, to observe and record patients' symptoms carefully for future generations. At the time, that was modern and revolutionary.

Also attributed to Hippocrates are the famous words: 'Let food be thy medicine and medicine be thy food.' He believed that eating certain foods would cure diseases. It hasn't turned out to be quite that easy, at least for chronic pain, but much good can be accomplished by eating sensibly. Scientific literature has quoted Hippocrates' statement often, although he apparently never said those words exactly. (He was of course not writing in English anyway.)

Why a person suffering from pain should eat (and drink) healthily

Many people with chronic pain have to not only cope with pain, but with fatigue, worries, mood swings, mobility problems, the side-effects of medications, impaired ability to work, and often financial hardship as well. In this situation, healthy eating isn't the first thing that comes to mind. On the contrary, many people seek comfort by feasting on rich foods and sweets. The powerful pleasurable experience produced by eating can be the only way to silence the inner accusatory voice – the voice that always repeats the same message that one really does not want to hear: 'You can't do anything to stop your pain; you are doomed.' However, there are several good reasons not to listen to that voice. First of all, you are not doomed. You can do many things to have better control over your pain. For example, instead of seeking quick comfort from eating, you can pay more attention to eating healthily. In the longer term, it will pay off.

Health trends and recommendations come and go, but I believe that now we truly are on the brink of a major scientific revolution – that's how startling the results of studies on the importance of the gut to human health are, for example. This statement does not refer only to the intestinal problems familiar to many chronic pain sufferers but, instead, to much more significant observations associated with neurological diseases, obesity, mental wellbeing, mood, and many other things, including pain.

What research tells us

Our intestines contain hundreds of billions of bacteria. Together, they weigh one and a half kilos – in fact, as much as our brain. Intestinal activity and cerebral activity are surprisingly similar to each other; for this reason the nervous system in the gut (the enteric nervous system) has even been referred to as the 'first brain' of early prehistoric mammals, based on evidence suggesting that it may have evolved before the actual brain. The intestines produce the same chemical neurotransmitters as our brain, but many times more – over 90 per cent of neurotransmitters are produced in the intestinal tract. These neurotransmitters strengthen, block or modify electronic and chemical messages between neurons (specialised nerve cells) and other cells. The intestines contain over 100 million neurons, which is much more than in the peripheral nervous system or the spinal cord. The brain of course is the neural centre, with 100 billion neurons. It and the gut influence and control each other, but both also act independently.

The gut differs from the brain in that it contains an enormous number of bacteria. However, it seems that even a healthy human brain contains some bacteria, though significantly fewer than the intestines. This, by the way, is a recent observation detected in research. It has traditionally been thought that the brain is a bacteria-free zone, but recent findings suggest that this is not the case. The role of bacteria in the brain isn't yet understood.

If a pathologist were to open and straighten an adult's intestines – including all of the intestinal villi and projections – and then spread it out to form a continuous 'cloth', it would cover the area of at least one tennis court. However, what is impressive is not only the area, but the quantity and diversity of microbes (bacteria, fungi, viruses etc.) in the intestines, especially in the large intestine. The large bowel provides a romping ground for trillions of microbes. The intestines have their own ecosystem; a system that differs from one person to the next. For example, the intestines of a slim person resemble a healthy woodland, with many different animals and plant species growing vibrantly in the rich soil. By contrast, the intestines of an obese person or, for example, a person with chronic fatigue syndrome, resemble an over-used lake where the animal population has declined and only a few plant species dominate; such a gut clearly has poorer microbes in terms of both quantity and quality.

Intestinal microbes play an important part in lipid (fat) metabolism: they affect, among other things, the regulation of fat storage, the balancing of blood sugar levels, the absorption of nutrients, and the way a person responds to hunger and satiation hormones. There have already been some preliminary studies where a procedure known as 'faecal microbiota transplant' has been used to introduce intestinal bacterial flora from healthy, slim people to overweight people, who have then lost weight. We still need more studies to find out how people might really benefit from such a procedure, which microbes are particularly beneficial and who should not have it because of possible side-effects.

Most intestinal bacteria are both useful and, indeed, necessary. Depletion of good bacteria and disturbance of their function increase the risk of illness. Recent studies have linked these disturbances with, among other things, depression, autism, severe stress, and many other symptoms and diseases traditionally considered to be 'of brain origin'. Bacteria themselves most likely aren't the cause of these conditions; rather, they contribute to their development.

Studies have shown that people with chronic pain, such as migraine, also have irritable bowel syndrome (IBS), coeliac disease, or an inflammatory bowel disease (IBD), such as Crohn's disease, more often than average. There are indications that the permeability of the intestines changes in people with these conditions, or simply with prolonged stress. The intestinal wall begins to 'leak', in which case intestinal bacteria and harmful molecules pass from the intestines into the bloodstream. Inflammation can be detected in the intestines, and a state of 'dysbiosis' sets in. Nutrients are absorbed poorly.

Probiotics, or 'good bacteria', are helpful in decreasing intestinal inflammation, correcting the dysfunction in the gut lining, and down-regulating hypersensitivity reactions. Accordingly, they reduce the effects of stress, and possibly even the effects of chronic pain. In the future, probiotics such as lactobacilli and bifidobacteria will probably be a part of modern pain management. There are already some indications of how they can be used – for instance, to alleviate the inflammation of rheumatoid arthritis, fatigue, depression and even social withdrawal. One interesting study showed that the consumption of probiotics for four weeks decreased the tendency to focus on thoughts that provoke negative emotions. The life of many chronic pain sufferers would be eased if their thoughts could more easily be shifted to positive things in place of worries and distress.

I will now go through those nutrients, foods and diets for which the most research data have accumulated in relation to pain management.

Omega-3 fatty acids

Omega-3 fatty acids, which are found particularly in fish oil but also in some plants (e.g. linseed) and grass-fed meat, have anti-inflammatory effects, so they are particularly suitable for pain states in which inflammation plays an important role. One of these is rheumatoid arthritis. Compared with people who do not eat fish, those who consume it one to three times a week have a 20–24 per cent lower risk of contracting rheumatoid arthritis. This is a significant reduction and an important finding, especially if rheumatoid arthritis runs in the family.

The consumption of fish oil is also beneficial against headache. In 2013 the journal *Pain*, the most prestigious scientific publication in the field of pain, published a high-quality study in which the amount of omega-6 fatty acids in the diet (from grains, seeds and factory-farmed meat) of chronic headache sufferers was reduced while the amount of omega-3 fatty acids was increased. The results were impressive: the number of hours spent suffering from headache in a day decreased, as did the number of headache days, and the quality of life increased significantly. In many studies, omega-3 has alleviated pain also in degenerative arthritis, irritable bowel syndrome, and menstruation. A suitable ratio of omega-3 to omega-6 fatty acids (1:3 or even 1:1) seems to accelerate the healing of nerve damage and intensify the functioning of the body's own pain relief system. Mood, alertness, memory and blood sugar balance – these also benefit from fish oils. Omega-3 fatty acids are obtained best from fatty fish such as salmon, mackerel and herring and from some nuts, especially walnuts (brain-like in appearance). And from a pill bottle, of course. The recommended daily dose of omega-3 is 2–3 grams per day.

Turmeric

According to a review of the ginger family of plants (Zingiberaceae) published in 2015, these plants can bring significant relief in chronic pain. In particular, turmeric has proved to be effective in treating pain and depression. According to a good-quality study, pain after gallbladder surgery, as well as the need for painkillers and fatigue, were decreased by the ingestion of turmeric. Some of the effects stem from the alleviation of inflammation. Turmeric appears to be a safer option than non-steroidal anti-inflammatory drugs (NSAIDs). It may also eases depression, which is – as I have said throughout the book – quite a common problem among pain sufferers. A minor difficulty associated with turmeric is that its use to season food is hardly adequate to yield substantial health benefits. For this reason, it is now sold in capsules – and even in this form, quite a few capsules need to be taken per day to get the promised benefits: 400 mg of turmeric is probably comparable to 200–400 milligrams of ibuprofen.

Other herbs and spices

A noteworthy amount of research data on other herbs and spices has also begun to accumulate. There is reasonably convincing scientific evidence about feverfew (*Tanacetum parthenium*), indicating that it prevents migraine attacks in some patients. For back pain, in turn, a skin cream containing the bell pepper *Capsicum frutescens* appears to be effective. Arnica gel seems to alleviate osteoarthritic pain, as does comfrey. The data on these plants available to date are based on publications produced by the prestigious international Cochrane Research Network. All available research data are compiled in the Cochrane Reviews, and the information obtained from the publications is considered to be reliable. More knowledge is sure to be gained in the coming years as researchers' interest in these non-pharmaceutical treatments has increased recently.

Caffeine

Many studies have been done on the use of caffeine for pain relief. A review of these studies, which included 20 of the best-quality studies, was published in 2014. These studies involved more than 7000 people. Combining the amount of caffeine present in one cup of coffee with ordinary analgesics, such as ibuprofen or paracetamol, gave better pain relief than taking the drug without caffeine. The effect was not very strong, as only about every tenth pain sufferer received a clear benefit from caffeine. Similar results were obtained in a second literature review which, however, only focused on headache patients.

However, be careful about drinking coffee and tea if you have sleep problems. A good night's sleep is much more important for pain relief than caffeine. If painkillers and coffee cause stomach irritation, forget about coffee or, if necessary, take medication to protect the stomach lining.

Chilli peppers

Chilli peppers are an interesting new analgesic. Studies have found that the chemical capsaicin found in them is effective, especially in treating neuropathic pain states where, in certain areas, even skin touch is perceived as pain. This sensitivity to touch may persist, for instance, after shingles. At its worst, even a quick light brush of the skin evokes pain. When a capsaicin patch or cream is applied to the skin, the skin begins to burn and swell for a moment. Capsaicin binds to the nociceptors that sense pain and heat. The strong burning sensation it provokes disturbs the nociceptors of the skin, and the skin's sensitivity to pain is reduced. The effect may become permanent if capsaicin is used an adequate number of times.

Vitamin D

Vitamin D from the diet or as a supplement is needed during the autumn and winter, because the sun, its natural source, isn't strong enough for the body to produce vitamin D. Vitamin D seems to have a number of positive effects, among others on the body's defence system and the functioning of the nervous system. Vitamin D deficiency is associated with skeletal diseases such as osteoporosis, and with diabetes, heart disease and vascular disease. Chronic pain patients often have a reduced level of vitamin D in the body. According to a study published by the esteemed Mayo Clinic in the United States, chronic pain patients whose level of vitamin D was too low used double the amount of strong painkillers when compared with chronic pain patients who had an adequate level of vitamin D. However, these studies don't indicate which is the cause and which the effect – the pain or the vitamin D deficiency.

It may even be that difficult pain restricts movement and increases staying indoors, which in turn leads to reduced exposure to the sun and consequently less vitamin D production. So far, international research data have not been able to show convincingly that chronic pain could be reduced by taking vitamin D. This was concluded in a systematic Cochrane Review of the research literature in 2015. However, since then a small but well-conducted study has been published in which vitamin D brought about a reduction in the pain and fatigue associated with fibromyalgia.

Vitamin C

Vitamin C may be helpful in pain management in at least migraine and complex regional pain syndrome (CRPS). In one study, a 500 mg daily dose of vitamin C for 50 days prevented the occurrence of CRPS. CRPS is a truly difficult chronic pain condition that usually occurs in a limb. It can start from a relatively small injury or fracture – sometimes a mere plaster of Paris cast can trigger CRPS.

According to at least one good-quality study, taking vitamin C before surgery would seem to reduce the need for a strong analgesic afterwards. Vitamin C has many different functions in the body. Its antioxidant properties may be especially significant with regard to pain. It prevents the oxidation of certain chemical compounds.

These compounds, or free radicals, can cause many types of damage in the body, among others by breaking cell membranes.

B vitamins and ubiquinol

There are indications that ubiquinone, at a daily dose of 150–300 mg, would be effective in migraine attack prevention. The antioxidant properties of ubiquinone may inhibit cellular oxidative stress (cell imbalance) and the resulting inflammatory reaction. Research shows riboflavin, or vitamin B2, may reduce the number of migraine attacks. More scientific evidence is still needed to support the use of other B-vitamins or a combination of B vitamins (vitamin B complex) in managing chronic pain. There are some research data on the use of vitamin B12 and folic acid (vitamin B9) to treat the depression often associated with pain. Both are needed for the synthesis of serotonin and other neurotransmitters.

Magnesium

Magnesium has become one of the important minerals in pain management. In the nervous system, magnesium is essential in the function and coordination between the nerves and the muscles. Postoperative pain and the need for strong analgesics can be reduced by administering magnesium to patients before surgery. There is some scientific evidence suggesting that taking magnesium reduces fibromyalgic pain and the neuropathic pain associated with shingles. One study found that people with chronic back pain, some of whose symptoms were neurogenic, benefited from magnesium: A six-week therapeutic regimen relieved pain and improved the mobility of the back – and the results could still be seen six months later. According to a recent literature review, magnesium also appears effective in preventing migraine attacks. A good number of studies have shown that many chronic pain sufferers, including migraine patients, have relatively little magnesium in the body – the real magnesium content in the body, however, is difficult to measure accurately. It isn't yet possible to say if this lack of magnesium is a result of its excessive use in the body due, for example, to prolonged stress related to chronic pain, or if a long-term magnesium deficiency is an underlying and causal factor in pain. In any case, it pays to make sure that you get enough magnesium from food. A high magnesium content is found especially in nuts – such as cashews and almonds – and various seeds – such as sunflower seeds, pumpkin seeds and pine nuts. Magnesium is also obtained, for instance, from whole grains, fish, avocado, banana and dark chocolate.

Chronic pain sufferers probably have a greater need for magnesium than healthy people, who usually get enough magnesium to cover the minimum daily requirement from just over half a cup (60–70 g) of pumpkin seeds. It's good to remember that the stomach protection medications (such as omeprazole) often used with painkillers tend to slow down the absorption of magnesium.

Special diets

Irritable bowel syndrome (IBS) is a very common additional complaint among chronic pain sufferers. Flatulence and cramping abdominal pain are among the most unpleasant symptoms of this complaint. The gut hardly ever works normally; instead, it's either too sluggish or too loud. At times the belly becomes distended, as though a basketball has been swallowed. Many people with IBS have obtained relief by following the **FODMAP** diet. This means eliminating the carbohydrates that are particularly well liked by the bacteria of the colon but cause fermentation, which then leads to symptoms of pain and swelling. The FODMAP diet is quite tedious, so before starting it, you should consider whether you can cope with your current symptoms or whether you need to revamp your diet according to the instructions – and whether you can do so without additional stress.

For many with migraine, a **low-fat diet rich in fibre and vegetables** has proved to be an effective way to manage pain. In one approach, the blood levels of antibodies produced by various foods have been measured for migraine patients. On the basis of the results, the patients have then eliminated the foodstuffs causing antibodies from their diet. In this way, the number of days in pain has decreased by one-third. There is also preliminary scientific evidence that a **ketogenic diet** low in carbohydrates and protein, and where energy is derived mainly from fat, might be effective for some migraine patients.

In one small but moderately good-quality study, a **low-fat diet rich in vegetables** alleviated neuropathic pain caused by diabetes. The diet involved avoiding animal products, restricting the consumption of fat to 20–30 grams a day, and favouring vegetables and foods with a low glycaemic index (the change in blood glucose due to carbohydrates absorbed from food).

The greatest number of studies on diet have been done for rheumatoid arthritis. The effects of a vegetarian diet, the Mediterranean diet, fasting, and the elimination diet on arthritic pain have been studied. Although some rheumatoid patients have obtained relief from their symptoms by eating plant-based food, as yet the study results measured with pain scales have not been convincing. However, a good deal of scientific evidence measured with other indicators (inflammatory reactions, insulin, etc.) has accumulated; naturally these benefit pain sufferers, too. Studies show that the Nordic diet, consisting of fish, rapeseed oil, low-fat dairy products, leafy vegetables, root vegetables, berries and local fruits, also functions well.

A recent study published in the journal *Neuroscience* showed that short-term and long-term memory deteriorates and new learning becomes more difficult if a person consumes large amounts of sugar and fat. Eating foods rich in trans fat also increases anxiety and symptoms of depression. Excessive consumption of sweet food and drink, in turn, seems to reduce cognitive flexibility. For people with chronic pain, flexible thinking is a crucially important means of coping with their pain. It's worth holding on to flexible thinking, as I explain in Chapter 3, Discover the importance of positive thinking.

But avoid alcohol

It's both normal and understandable that sometimes people get the idea of using alcohol to relieve persistent pain. In fact, it's a surprisingly common form of self-medication: one in three people with chronic pain report using alcohol as an analgesic. It's true that a moderate amount of alcohol brings temporary pain relief. This has even been shown in experimental studies. However, alcohol shouldn't be considered a regular means of pain management. The unfortunate truth is that it causes more harm than good.

Dulling the pain with drink would require a great deal of wine, cider or beer. Of course, a small dose provides a brief relief from the annoyance of living with pain, but when, after a larger dose, the hangover sets in, there isn't a trace of pain relief. Instead, the entire body is sensitised to pain after an evening of drinking – in addition to the unrelenting throbbing of the head. Tippling in the evening also disturbs getting a good night's sleep, which is essential to anyone with chronic pain. Drinking even more increases anxiety and symptoms of depression.

What's more, alcohol can wash good management attempts down the drain, as it interferes with medical treatment for chronic pain. Moreover, painkillers and alcohol are not compatible. Adverse effects – gastric and intestinal bleeding and liver damage – often set in unnoticed. Opioid drugs strengthen the depressant effect of alcohol on the central nervous system. Opioids and spirits together induce respiratory depression, each year sending too many people too early to their grave. Moreover, spirits are a powerful chemical solvent, and abundant, prolonged consumption of alcohol is therefore known to cause destruction of thin nerve fibres, which is a nasty painful condition in itself.

Chapter 7

My own experience

A few years ago I listened to a neurologist's lecture on migraine. The neurologist mentioned the Chinese restaurant syndrome. I pricked up my ears. I then heard for the first time that a flavour-enhancer called monosodium glutamate (E621 or 'MSG') is added in particular to Asian foods with the purpose of producing a umami, or savoury, taste. Umami is the fifth basic taste – a pleasant savoury taste that arouses hunger. Unfortunately, monosodium glutamate can trigger a migraine attack if a person is hypersensitive to the additive. During that lecture, I understood that I am such a person. I had wondered why so often after eating at an Asian restaurant, my head began to ache in the same way as in a migraine attack, only the pain came much faster and more strongly than usual. I love Vietnamese food, but in my case, the price of a restaurant visit, aside from the bill, is an antimigraine pill.

The increased migraine sensitivity has weakened my capacity to tolerate alcohol, and with age it has fallen to almost nil. I am a bit annoyed about it, but I know that it's not the end of the world. Sparkling wine is a trendy drink, but for me it is one of the most horrible headache-provoking drinks. Red wine is nearly as bad. I can't even think about spirits, at least not whiskeys or cognac. Fortunately, my head can still withstand a few beers, but as soon as I have more than that, I need an antimigraine pill again.

I must admit that my sweet tooth screams for pick 'n' mix sweets. I also love high-fat cheeses. However, I feel better when I curb my intake of sugar and fat. I'm calmer, my ability to concentrate is better, and I feel a stronger sense of coping. When I eat sensibly, I have fewer guilty thoughts about actually having caused my pain myself through my bad eating habits.

What you can do – How you can eat better to manage your pain

- Draw up a concrete plan to use as a departure point and roadmap. Be committed to it. Don't try to change everything all at once; you'll be able to proceed further in small steps. If you decide to increase your vitamin D intake this week, you can add omega-3 to your programme next month. A discussion with a dietitian will help you to outline your eating and plan a diet that suits you.
- Many things that suit a particular person can only be found by trial and error. In general, the same programme should be continued for at least four to six weeks so that the effects can be seen. Getting used to a new taste requires 10–15 tasting sessions.
- You can't go very far wrong if you adopt a diet rich in berries, vegetables, other fruits, wholegrain fibre, nuts, fish, acidophilus products (probiotics) and fresh water. Make sure to get enough protein. Chicken, legumes and curd cheese are excellent sources for this.
- Many pain sufferers have reported being helped by omitting all added sugar and white flour from their diet. After managing to resist pasta, French bread and sweet buns for a couple of weeks, they begin to feel appreciably better. You can measure the effects, for instance by trying to manage in this way with a smaller dose of painkillers.
- An analgesic cream containing chilli to be applied locally on the skin of the painful area (at one's own risk) can be made at home. The instructions can be found from various sources online.
- Avoid natural products for which no reliable research data are available yet. Wait for further information. Liver

damage is a costly price to pay for impatience.
- It pays to protect the good bacteria of the gut and avoid unnecessary antibiotic treatments. Just one course of antibiotic treatment can upset the intestinal bacteria for one or even two years.
- Other good, reliable sources of information are: http://painconcern.org.uk/diet-and-pain/ and www.arthritisresearchuk.org/arthritis-information/hints-and-tips/diet/foods-to-avoid.asp

Chapter 8

Move that body

At the present time, it is difficult, if not impossible, to avoid hearing about the unbeatable benefits of physical exercise. Exercise is medicine, it is said. A great many health professionals swear that it is the **best** medicine. However, just as a good many of us do not take the pills doctors prescribe for us, many of us aren't physically active at all, or do very little. We all have our reasons for not exercising: bad weather, lack of time, no suitable workout gear... Lack of knowledge about the health benefits is hardly an obstacle given the present flood of information about them. Nor is there any lack of opportunity to exercise: in the UK as well as in most Western countries, there are plenty of inexpensive indoor exercise facilities, and parks, green areas, woodlands, fields and lakes available for outdoor activities. Lack of interest doesn't explain immobility either, as, when asked, only a small minority of people say they have no interest at all in physical activity.

The most important reason for lack of exercise seems to be failure to get going – an inability to find the motivation to get out on a bike or go to a gym or Pilates class. Gravity seems to weigh us down much more when it's time to leave for the gym or go for a jog. Our legs become as heavy as cement bags, and someone must have put the world's most powerful magnet under the sofa. It's still possible to raise your arm enough to fish for the remote control on the coffee table. An internal dialogue begins: I had such a hard day at work, and I ache all over. The weather is bad, too. What if I didn't go today; but go tomorrow instead...? The mind twists and turns, and not even a sense of guilt drives us to get moving.

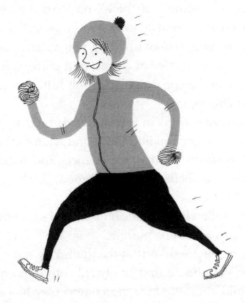

Another important reason for being passive is that we've learned to avoid physical activity when we have health problems. Many have had it drummed into their heads that feeling pain is a sign of danger, and anything that causes or worsens it must therefore be limited and avoided. Fear of worsening tissue damage or re-injury will make us squeeze the remote control even tighter and think: 'I will not move until I am completely pain-free.'

Why a person suffering from pain should be physically active

Earlier I explained how the brain tricks us by feeding us memories and meanings that aren't always true. As far as exercise is concerned, you can use the same tactics: you can mislead and deceive your brain in return. The deception works, you see, both ways: by feeding our brain a line, we can alter the default settings that prevent us from acting in a particular way.

We may have learned that there's no point to exercising if the heart isn't pounding and there's no sweating. No pain, no gain, as Jane Fonda famously put it. You may still remember the PE teacher from your school insisting you should exercise for at least 45 minutes or an hour at a time, and preferably every day. If you don't, you'll come down with self-inflicted illnesses and suffer a miserable fate.

Let's now learn to think in a new way: do only as much as you can, so long as you get moving. Enjoy and rejoice in what you do and feel like, reinforce positive experiences and good memories. Forget health and focus on feeling good. Trick yourself into doing it.

Try out the following and see how it works for you. Earlier in the day, you have perhaps planned to go for a walk or a run in the evening, or for a workout at the gym. When it comes to the time to leave, you should first gently rid your mind of its normal mumbling following about the hard day you've had at work and the many obstacles to exercising. Tell yourself that you'll first walk round the block and do your unfinished chores afterwards. If walking feels awful, then you can just come home. Or tell yourself that if you feel weighed down at the gym, you'll pedal on the exercise cycle bike for just five minutes and then leave. Or promise yourself that it's enough to do three short workouts on the floor, next to the sofa. If you feel up to doing more, that's great, but if not, that's fine, too.

Convince yourself in this way: the most important reason to go for a walk is that it's nice to be outside in the fresh air. It will make you happy. Your brain will get oxygen and your thinking will be sharper. On the other hand, the indoor air at the gym may not be the best, but if you lack the stamina to toil away, you may catch a glimpse of beautiful bodies. That will also make you feel good. Remind yourself of how much fun cycling is, whether you take it slowly on an old-fashioned bike or zip down the road on a new hybrid model. Either way, the legs pump wellbeing throughout the body.

Five to 10 minutes of physical exercise three times a week is enough at the start. Don't aim for more – especially if you haven't been active at all for a while. It's essential to teach your brain that physical activity is associated with feeling good. When you repeat this for a few weeks, your new mode of thinking will become automatic.

Remind yourself of a specific time (and there will be many!) when you've been able to be physically active and exercise but have hardly even noticed your pain. You may have been enjoying moving in great company. It's worth recalling these memories over and over again so that positive, real memories are reinforced, and painful, often distorted memories recede.

Walking round the block will become a longer walk without your noticing it, or doing three gymnastics exercises will feel so good that you'll want to do more. Hold on to the emotion that follows regular physical activity, filling both mind and body: the mild feeling of restlessness about wanting to be active once again today. It takes just two weeks to get hooked on physical activity. In this regard, being active outdoors is verifiably more effective than indoor exercise in developing this positive addiction.

What research tells us

Tolerating pain better

Being physically active is a great tool for pain management in that it influences many other tools in your pain management tool box. Exercising regularly improves your sleep at night, lifts your mood, decreases fatigue and increases energy levels. The feeling of being in control of your life increases, and you find that you're capable of many other things that used to seem difficult. An increased tolerance is, of course, essential with regard to pain.

If a person has chronic pain, the brain readily becomes

overprotective. But once you've learned that your chronic pain is no longer a sign of danger, you can safely allow yourself some physical activity despite slight pain.

In an Australian study, healthy young people who didn't go in for exercise were chosen as subjects. Their pain threshold and pain tolerance were measured before the study began. 'Pain threshold' refers to the lowest strength of an external stimulus that is sensed as pain. It indicates the moment when you feel as though you can 'hear' the pain but can still tolerate it. Pain tolerance, in turn, indicates the greatest amount of a pain-inducing stimulus that a person can stand. When you put one of your hands in very cold water, in a few seconds you begin to feel pain (pain threshold), but you can still keep your hand in the water until 'aaargh...' you have to take it out (pain tolerance).

After the pain threshold measurements were made, half of the subjects continued their passive life as usual. The other half started to do physical exercise. The exercise was simple and fairly short in duration: they had to pedal an exercise bike for half an hour three times a week. The pedalling resistance was raised each week, but the time on the bike remained the same.

The study lasted for six weeks. As expected, the physical performance capacity of the group that cycled on the exercise bike improved during that time. The purpose of the study, however, was to test whether such a very moderate amount of exercise affected the participants' pain threshold or pain tolerance, which were measured again at the end of the study.

The results were interesting. There were no changes in the pain threshold of either the group whose members had pedalled on the exercise bike or the group whose members had led a passive life. However, the subjects who had pedalled on the exercise bike had better tolerance for the feeling of pain than before. This correlated with the increase in physical fitness: subjects whose physical fitness had increased the most during the study also had the greatest improvement in pain tolerance.

According to the researchers, this isn't merely a reflection of physical changes in the body. It is probably that, thanks to physical exercise, the brain begins to see the person as a 'tough guy' – as someone 'tougher' than the person thought him/herself to be. The brain allows us to continue for a long time despite the pain, since the pain is no longer frightening – even if its intensity hasn't weakened. It's simply experienced as more tolerable.

Pain tolerance is affected by many things, such as the nature of the pain. This also affects the type of assistance being physically active can provide. Many people with chronic back pain, rheumatoid arthritis, shoulder pain, or hip or knee osteoarthritis experience significant pain relief when they regularly engage in brisk physical exercise. Its effectiveness is of the same order as non-steroidal anti-inflammatory drugs (NSAIDs). Exercise strengthens the spine, muscles and tendons, and increases their flexibility. It is also beneficial for posture control. In the brain and central nervous system, exercise enhances the brain's own production of painkillers, that is, opioids and endorphins. It also enhances the function of neurotransmitters and the so-called descending nerve pathways that inhibit pain. In addition, exercise alleviates the inflammatory reactions of the body.

Have fun taking exercise

There are many people, however, for whom exercise doesn't work in this way. In so-called 'central sensitisation', as in fibromyalgia, the central nervous system maintains pain; then, physical activity doesn't activate the body's own pain regulation systems because there is a disturbance in the system. A normal physical exercise class or workout at the gym may make the body ache for a couple of days or a week, causing the motivation to keep exercising to dissipate. However, physical activity is a prerequisite for wellbeing among these pain patients, too, but the dose needs to adjusted so that it's quite small at first. Sometimes 10 to 15 minutes of walking, aqua-jogging or Pilates is enough. The time can be extended gradually, say, at three-monthly intervals. It will be so much easier to cope with the pain if you teach yourself to do physical activities that you enjoy and accept that the pain may even be a little worse initially, but it does not indicate harm or danger.

Perhaps surprisingly, many adults with chronic pain have been physically active as children and young people; they've often been very sporty and enjoyed being active. To them, sport as a hobby has been a precondition of their wellbeing. Studies show that if a person has to decrease his/her activity when young – and especially if their quality of sleep begins to suffer in consequence – many will develop widespread pain as an adult. Among these young people, research has found a disturbance in the body's stress mechanism, in what is known as the hypothalamic-pituitary-adrenal (HPA) axis, as well as changes in immune response and autonomic functions. In some people, the body thus responds to **lack of exercise** with pain throughout the body.

According to studies, muscle condition among women suffering from widespread pain is on average 40 per cent worse than that of healthy women of the same age. If you have pain and stop exercising, then your muscles will atrophy. People with fibromyalgia show changes in their bodies that promote this kind of muscle loss: microscopic changes take place in muscle fibres, and the neuromuscular system is no longer able to maintain motor control in the same way as before. Muscular blood flow is weakened, and the muscles suffer from oxygen deficiency. The changes are also linked with tissue growth and repair mechanisms and with energy metabolism. All is not lost, however. Fibromyalgic pain can also be reduced by physical exercise, especially by determined muscle strength training. Even accepting pain becomes easier with exercising.

Neck pain and tension headache are very common complaints. They can be effectively alleviated, and the use of analgesics reduced, by isometric exercises that improve the strength of the neck muscles. First, one needs to learn to control the position of the head. After that, tightening the muscles of the neck is practised against one's own hand as resistance. Finally, the muscles are trained against an elastic band as resistance. According to current knowledge, aerobic endurance training can also provide slight relief for pain in the neck and shoulder region. Mere stretching seems to have a rather modest effect.

Find your own sport

Many exercise modes are well suited to chronic pain patients. Water sports (aqua jogging, water aerobics, swimming) are especially recommended. It does the chronic pain patient good to be in water and exercise against its soft resistance. Water pressure causes the activation of subcutaneous neurofibrilli (minute nerve fibres under the skin), which in turn intensifies the pain relief mechanisms of the central nervous system. Pampering oneself with a bath or a visit to a spa is also good for treating pain. (For more about this see Chapter 5, Do what you enjoy.)

Walking helps relieve chronic pain and improves functioning. A recently published review and meta-analysis collected the research results of almost 20 studies and, on this basis, found that the relief for chronic pain obtained by walking, at best, is moderate, that is, of the same order as analgesics. Another review showed that walking improves pain, disability, quality of life and fear-avoidance among people with chronic low back pain. Walking is free and can be done anywhere and in any way: with or without Nordic walking poles; alone or with others; in the countryside or the city... Many American shopping malls open their doors early, long before the shops, so that people can walk there. Groups of people doing power walking, which is a faster-paced type of fitness walking, can be seen in these locations. They are a good place to go for a walk, as the temperature is usually pleasant (often air-conditioned) and toilets and water fountains are close by. Equally, there aren't many alternatives, as in the United States the roads usually have no pavement.

If you want to improve your physical fitness, you may have read from the internet or a magazine that you should take at least 10,000 steps a day. And if you want to keep your weight in check, 12,000 steps a day are required, and 16,000 if you want to lose weight. I have to say that for someone with chronic pain (like myself), these are rather tough targets.

Fortunately, recent studies have made the targets more reasonable, making them more suitable for chronic pain patients. For a person with osteoarthritic knee pain, 6000 steps a day is enough to maintain good functioning. This amount means an hour of uninterrupted walking at a brisk pace averaging 100 steps per minute – or, at a slower pace, 60 steps per minute for an hour and 40 minutes. This figure includes all of the day's steps. For a person with fibromyalgia, 5000 steps a day already improves pain management. This is only about 1000 to 2000 steps more than the average person with fibromyalgia walks in a day. A good rule of thumb is: 15 minutes of walking equals about 1000 steps. An additional 15 minutes of movement per day is thus a major benefit for a person with chronic pain. If you reach 5000 to 7500 steps a day on a regular basis, you can be satisfied. The better your mood when you walk, the more you will benefit from this activity when it comes to managing your pain.

Pilates has been scientifically proved to be helpful for lower back pain. In 2015 the famous Cochrane Review Group published a review that focused on some 500 patients with chronic lower back pain. The review concluded that there is moderate evidence that the Pilates method helps to relieve pain and improve function. Pilates is not superior to other types of exercise, but the results of the review encourage us to try. Pilates is a calm exercise mode that teaches body management and breathing techniques while also strengthening the mid-body muscles in particular.

Some interesting scientific evidence has accumulated on T'ai chi indicating that this exercise method alleviates pain and improves functioning, especially among low back pain and osteoarthritis patients. In addition, mood improves, stress and anxiety are relieved, and confidence in one's own physical mobility is reinforced. T'ai chi is a Chinese exercise method that combines meditation with slow, soft movement. Series of moves differing in length are carried out while simultaneously concentrating on breathing. More advanced users can add speed and physically more demanding exercises. T'ai chi develops muscle tone, muscle and joint flexibility, coordination and balance, and generates peace of mind.

My own experience

When it comes to physical activity especially, I've had to adapt my life to my pain symptoms. As a young person, I competed in team handball at a national level, and I've always been very active. In recent years, I've had to give up rapid-paced physical activity, including all the ball games that I particularly enjoyed in the past. I've both mourned and cursed this loss, but I haven't got hung up on those feelings. New activities – biking, aquajogging, and Pilates – are more suitable for an aching body, although at times the tempo is too relaxed for me. However, I can get a sense of the speed of physical activity through visualisation exercises and music.

I have found that my brain, overly attuned to pain, can be surprisingly inventive at making me passive: as my pain increased over time a variety of reasons for staying put seemed ever more justified. Eventually, I tired of listening to my inner voice repeating excuses for doing nothing, like bad weather and lack of time, and I solved the problem by acquiring a second-hand exercise bike, which I stationed on my glazed-in balcony. Even a freezing temperature doesn't bother me as I pedal away, woolly cap on my head, working up a sweat while Pink, or the Bee Gees, sets the pace. (There's no way I could pedal for more than five minutes without music.) Just 30 minutes of biking, changing the resistance as I cycle, meets the day's need for exercise. On many occasions while tying the laces of my trainers, I've told myself that I'll stop after five minutes if pedalling gets just too boring. But I've always continued for longer than that.

Another new favourite activity is aquajogging. I regularly go to my local swimming pool and do this activity for 30-45 minutes. Aquajogging is like slowly running in the water wearing a flotation device (belt) around your waist. Your feet are not supposed to touch the bottom of the pool, so I do it at the deep end. Aquajogging has recently gained popularity in many countries. To be honest, for me, it seemed rather boring initially, until I came up with the idea that I could do some deep thinking at the same time. I do a visualisation exercise called 'What will I be doing 15 years from now?' In my visualisation I transport myself from my hometown's public swimming pool to the pool of a large Spanish villa on the beach of the Mediterranean Sea. Never a cloud in the sky there. How wonderfully the light breeze brushes my face. Sometimes, in my mind, I do my aquajogging in the rooftop pool of a Manhattan skyscraper and consider my life from a bird's eye view. It's easy to fill those 30 to 45 minutes in this way.

Following a long break, swimming has started to go well for me. Some years ago, the sideways kick of the breaststroke felt unpleasant to my operated-on knee, so I started to think that knee pain would always prevent me from swimming. And I stopped. A typical situation: once you've fixed a conclusion in your mind, such as 'I'll never be able to swim again', it becomes something that you don't even attempt – a self-fulfilling prophecy. A few years ago, on a holiday trip to Spain I had to try swimming because aquajogging wasn't possible, as the water level in the pool was too low, and I wanted to get some exercise in the water anyway. Swimming went well and I got enthusiastic about it again, especially when a swimmer friend taught me a little about technique. Swimming brings a welcome change to aquajogging.

Studies have repeatedly shown that exercise and good fitness don't provide full protection against pain. Pain symptoms occur among both the physically active and the couch potatoes. In my own work I've found, however, that exercise helps pain sufferers to cope with the symptoms, and research confirms this. Of all my patients with chronic pain, it seems that those who maintain an active lifestyle are the ones who manage best. They are able to exercise and be generally active despite the pain. With regard to quality of life and optimism, they are in a class of their own.

What you can do

- Go in for types of sport and exercise that you like, but if the more gruelling types repeatedly cause soreness, try something lighter. Learn to be flexible and allow yourself to consider your health. If you can't do Pilates or a particular movement at your yoga class, you can do an easier version or some other movement. Instructors will often offer options without asking, or on request. If an online exercise video instructs you to run in place and you can't do it, march in place at a brisk pace instead.
- Learn new routines; for instance, stand while watching the evening news. Even 15 minutes of standing, as a break from a longer spell of sitting, brings significant health effects. You can do light gymnastics exercises or pedal on an exercise bike at the same time.
- Draw up a concrete, simple and realistic set of targets for yourself: what you want to achieve, in what time, and what you intend to do to reach your goal. You can ask for help from a professional, such as a sports instructor, personal trainer or physiotherapist. Keep a diary of your actions. Try also to record your physical feelings and emotions before exercising and about half an hour afterwards.
- Pack a sports bag with your kit or gym gear in the evening, and place it by the front door. Or place the clothes for your morning jog or walk next to your bed, with your alarm

clock partially under the clothes. That way, it will be easier to put the clothes on.

- Many experience a lack of motivation after two or three weeks. Should this occur, add something nice to your physical activity: music, new workout clothes, a new sport, good company. Being physically active together increases the feeling of wellbeing more than exercising alone.

- Praise yourself after each exercise session, and glow with enthusiasm about your achievement. This will strengthen your brain's reward system and lower the threshold to be active another time.

- Don't worry if you've had a few weeks' break. It's not dangerous to stop and start again. Tell yourself that you'll go next time, but don't throw in the towel altogether.

- Clear away obstacles to physical activity from your daily life. Go to the gym or for a swim straight from work. Take advantage of the sports facilities near your home. You can do a lot at home, and the internet is full of videos on gymnastics, yoga and dance. Consoles also feature some fun sport games to play.

- Go dancing, join a rowing team or your neighbourhood football team. Invite your friends or neighbours to go for a walk with you.

- Be bold and try new types of sport: T'ai chi, frisbee golf, standup paddleboarding or curling. Enjoy physical activity and movement.

- More information can be found on the internet, for instance at: www.nhs.uk/live-well/exercise/free-fitness-ideas/ or www.nhs.uk/oneyou/be-healthier/move-more/

Chapter 9

Experience the power of mindfulness

Tens of thousands of thoughts whirl through our heads during the day. They can't be controlled, they come and go. Even while reading this, your thoughts are momentarily floating away to other things. The more tired you are, the more easily your mind begins to wander. You may contemplate what dish to make in the evening. You intermittently recall last weekend's events or yesterday's phone call with your ageing mother. Maybe you wonder how your knee pain will withstand tomorrow's Zumba class.

More than 90 per cent of our daily thoughts are just like this: they jump to the future or slide back to the past without our noticing. We can't influence either the future or the past, yet in our thoughts we spend most of our time in one or the other. Only every tenth thought of the day concerns the moment we live in.

Mindfulness is a form of meditation where we learn an open, curious and accepting attitude towards ourselves, the events of our life, and the emotions we experience. It has evolved from Buddhist tradition, but in its present form it isn't associated with anything religious.

During mindfulness exercises, a person learns to focus their attention on things that are happening at that moment without trying to evaluate or change their course. The sensations of the body, too, can be learned only by acknowledging and accepting them, even if they cause unpleasant feelings. Even difficult emotions need not be repelled or suppressed. By increasing our presence in the here and now, with time we can begin to feel better both mentally and physically.

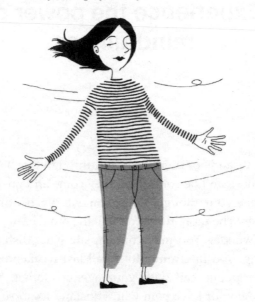

Why a person suffering from pain should practise mindfulness

Mindfulness has been used mainly as a relaxation and stress management method, but today it also has a role in pain management. At the beginning of the book, I explained how the cerebral cortex of many chronic pain sufferers is subject to constant activity, a kind of chaotic flurry of electric nerve signals. The central nervous system is in a sensitised state and the pain regulation system is disturbed.

Through meditation and mindfulness exercises, this excessive irritability can be calmed down. In addition, the ability to observe and interpret the body's signals becomes more meaningful. It is easier to manage and regulate habits when the automatic functions obsessively seeking pleasure no longer guide us. Pain may have caused a person to seek comfort, for instance, from eating. With the help of mindfulness, we have the chance to stop and get rid of the need to struggle or flee, to which we have been driven by pain. The power of our emotions decreases, our mind calms down, our body relaxes, and sleep improves.

Increasing mindfulness and acceptance doesn't mean that pain must be tolerated just by gritting one's teeth. Mindfulness makes it possible to break the vicious cycle of denial, rejection and avoidance and instead to gain a more compassionate and more accepting attitude towards bodily sensations and the feelings and thoughts they cause.

Meditation is easy to implement, it is inexpensive or at best even free, and it has very few if any adverse effects. It is one of the safest and simplest ways to improve pain management. But at the outset it requires learning and practising and, after the beginning, constant maintenance in order to keep up the skill.

What research tells us

So many individual studies on mindfulness in pain management have accumulated in the past 10 years that it has already been possible to conduct systematic reviews. Individual studies have been quite small and their quality hasn't always been very high, for which reasons convincing scientific evidence for mindfulness directly and significantly reducing chronic pain intensity is lacking. However, research has shown promising results with regard to increasing acceptance of pain and coping with it. It becomes easier to face adverse events. Also, quite convincing evidence exists for the effects of mindfulness on reducing many of the co-occurring symptoms related to chronic pain – that is, stress, sleep problems, anxiety and depression. I do therefore recommend trying it out as an additional pain treatment – as one more tool in the pain management tool box. It is easy to implement and does not cost anything.

A systematic review published in 2017 in the *Annals of Behavioural Medicine* synthesised evidence for the efficacy and safety of mindfulness meditation interventions in treating chronic pain in adults. According to the 38 randomised comparative studies included in the review, mindfulness meditation slightly improves pain and depression symptoms and quality of life. Randomised comparative studies are considered in science to be the most credible form of research study. Another recent review indicated that mindfulness also reduced the feeling of being weighed down by pain. Mindfulness has also been shown to help sufferers accept pain. A review from 2019 showed that learning mindfulness skills in a group is also a potentially helpful way to improve chronic pain management.

The most interesting new research results relate to changes observed in the brain and the extinction of the body's inflammatory reactions. It seems that practising mindfulness skills produces wide brain-level changes. It has been possible to visualise changes in areas of the brain involved in the regulation of feelings, mood, self-image and behaviour, as well as in the sensation of pain. There is even evidence that in some areas of the brain, meditation slows the development of age-related structural changes and thus contributes to the preservation of memory and other cognitive functions. Also, the effect of mindfulness on increasing the blood level of telomerase, an enzyme that slows ageing, has been demonstrated, as has the alleviation of inflammatory reactions in the body. Research on mindfulness as a complementary mode of treatment for other chronic diseases, such as asthma, diabetes, cardiovascular disease and inflammatory bowel disease (IBD), has therefore begun.

By learning how to be consciously present in the moment, it is possible to give up strong analgesics or gain better control over their use. In an American study, 115 chronic pain patients were randomly divided into two groups: every day, one group performed 15 minutes of mindfulness exercises with a CD and three minutes of respiratory exercises before taking their daily dose of opioid, a strong analgesic medication. The second group received peer support before taking their daily medication.

Among the patients in the meditation group, the need for strong analgesic medication fell by 63 per cent while the reduction among those in the peer support group was 32 per cent. After the study, those in the meditation group coped with pain better. They also learned to adopt a more peaceful attitude and to react more calmly to pain symptoms. The positive effect lasted at least to the end of the three-month follow-up period.

My own experience

Despite my outward appearance of calm, I have a somewhat restless soul. I get easily enthused, and I contemplate and plan the future energetically. I rarely brood over the past, but I do catch myself at it from time to time. When I began to pay attention to the matter, I found myself mentally present sadly very little during my free time. I think my work is at least partly to blame. I always try to be intently present with my patients. Patient work is quite intense, and it also uses a lot of energy. Thus I've noticed that I want to let my thoughts fly in all directions during my free time. I'm unable to focus on listening or making precise observations about my surroundings. Reading a paper is easily interrupted, as I have to check my emails and think about other things. From time to time, even my own children point out – with reason: 'Mother, why aren't you listening... again?'

Eventually, I decided to turn over a new leaf and learn the skill of being present during my free time. I was also interested in trying whether I could obtain relief from my pain symptoms by being present consciously. I took part for one autumn in a mindfulness course at an adult education institute and learned an attitude of acceptance towards myself and my feelings. I learned to observe my environment and to use my senses more. I learned a self-made mantra: smell, taste, sense, look, hear, feel.

When walking my dog on the city streets, I started to look again at the beautiful shapes of the buildings and the colours of the environment. I noticed how the sea sparkled brightly and the rays of sunshine were beautifully reflected from the window of an old building. The smell of autumn wafted through the city, the tramcars clattered cheerfully, and the speakers of the food shop emitted good music! Now I try to stop to sample tastes and to focus on how the water flowing in the shower feels on my skin.

I began to practise stopping my thoughts, slowing down to observe my breathing. Nowadays I may do so for a few minutes at my desk with my eyes closed. Sometimes I pay attention to my breathing when in the underground, sometimes on the sofa at home. I find that this exercise works every time. I feel how my mind calms down, how I relax, and my brain fog clears. I feel then that I can cope with my pain better, because I'm calmer. But during the hurry of everyday life these skills are often forgotten and there are days when it is as if patches cover my eyes and earplugs block my ears. Eating again becomes fast-paced hunger satisfaction, the shower is just a routine, and pain takes over my thoughts... For this reason, the calendar on my mobile phone has an alarm that every couple of weeks reminds me: Helena, your life is here and now. You should be here too.

What you can do

- Look into options for mindfulness training – for instance, at your local adult education institute or library or community centre.
- Many work places have mindfulness groups organised by occupational health services or the firm's HR department. Ask your HR department about this or suggest they set up a group.
- It's also possible to dive into the world of meditation through self-learning. On the internet, search for the word 'mindfulness' or 'meditation'. Numerous smartphone applications have also been developed for daily use.
- Plenty of books and CDs are available in libraries and

shops. The developer and best known advocate of mindfulness is Jon Kabat Zinn, an American; his books can be found in many shops and online. British-American comedian Ruby Wax has spoken and written about mindfulness and is worth checking out.
- Visit the mindful pages of the NHS www.nhs.uk/conditions/stress-anxiety-depression/mindfulness/ or www.mindful.org/

Chapter 10

Keep working – don't give up

People suffering from chronic pain end up on sick leave and Statutory Sick Pay (SSP) significantly more often than others. Pain symptoms cause a startling number of days of sick leave in most Western countries. Around 25 per cent of chronic pain patients lose their jobs. It has been estimated that the costs of chronic pain are higher than those of diabetes, cardiovascular disease and cancer combined. Work disability is a major reason for these enormous sums related to chronic pain.

One reason for this epidemic of work disability is that a lot of outdated ideas, attitudes and beliefs associated with pain still prevail in the work place, healthcare services and legislation. The fresh winds blowing in pain research have brought a new view of pain but things have not yet changed enough. It is time to open the window to new thinking.

Why a person living with pain should work

Every fifth adult suffers from chronic pain. Many of these people go to work with their pain symptoms. Many of them are lucky because their work conditions can be and have been modified so that they can cope. They can manage also because they have decided to cope. They don't give in to pain nor do they allow it to take valuable things away from their life, such as the enjoyment of working and an adequate livelihood. For many living with

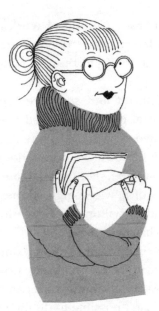

chronic pain, work is a source of wellbeing – it satisfies some of their deepest needs: life has meaning and purpose; they can feel useful and fulfilled and use their know-how and experience; and they can belong to a community.

Social interaction and the work environment may have an even greater significance than we realise. A good team, in which co-workers encourage one another and help each other out, supports coping at work. In these circumstances, it's good to go to the workplace in the morning because there we encounter friendly people and hear interesting stories. Our line manager, if available and understanding, also has a central role. With the manager's help, tasks can be tailored so that working is possible despite pain.

The 'lucky ones' also include those whose occupational healthcare service (if they have access to one) actively supports coping at work and provides versatile, rehabilitative support measures. Modern healthcare takes, or should take, a comprehensive approach to the individual, and his/her health problems. Conserving resources is at least as important as screening for diseases. Coping at work is also made more possible by an understanding and encouraging family. With their help, life can continue to be rewarding and meaningful despite pain.

Working is a difficult and sensitive topic for many with chronic pain, as it is also for their loved ones, co-workers and bosses. It is associated with surprisingly strong emotions. The topic is also difficult for me as an occupational health physician and chronic pain sufferer. However, I am bolstered by the comforting findings of new research studies and by the belief that new understanding will make the world a kinder place for people living with chronic pain.

The issues I discuss in this chapter don't mean that you would not have the right to be absent from work whenever illness so requires. Everyone living with chronic pain sometimes has periods when it isn't possible to do their job. At such times, the only solution may be to stay away from work for a while – or leave the job completely, if the situation is very difficult. However, no stone should be left unturned before anyone with chronic pain is allowed to be excluded from working life permanently. This means all options need to be looked at for ways to continue working and ways to manage pain effectively – not just painkillers, sick leave and surgery.

What does research tell us?

All over the world, there are many success stories about healthy workplaces where people with chronic pain can keep working. These prime examples show that working methods, tasks, tools, working hours, management and the physical and mental work environment can be developed and tailored, as long as there is courage and the will to succeed – and a common mission. These companies and work communities have decided to ban thinking along the lines that 'This work can't be adapted or modified.' They have creatively considered what kinds of work/tasks the company needs done and how these things can be achieved differently.

'All workplaces are full of work that no one has time to do, needing someone to do it,' said an HR supervisor at one of these companies. Meaningful work has been found within these companies for people who, despite various attempts, haven't been able to continue in their former jobs. The new work isn't necessarily the same as what they were originally hired to do, but it's still a job that has made it possible to maintain their ability to work and support a good quality of life, and financial security. Thanks to these active efforts, other workers in these organisations have also started to feel better and take more pleasure in their work. Sick leave has decreased considerably; productivity has risen; and staff turnover has declined. What's more, the companies concerned have saved millions.

According to current understanding, continuing working, even if only part-time, is rehabilitating to people with chronic pain. It usually isn't necessary to wait for complete relief from pain before returning to work – nor is it even possible for a person with chronic pain to be totally pain-free, at least not for long periods of time. I know this may seem like a strange idea to some people. We have had the idea drummed into our heads that pain is always a sign of danger and working while in pain will lead to worsening of tissue damage and, in the worst case scenario, to disability. This is one of our society's deeply rooted myths. Continuing in a suitable job despite some pain rarely causes permanent damage in the painful tissues, whereas fear and worry about the danger of pain often cause people more harm. Pain isn't always the main cause of incapacity to work. Lack of strength and fatigue associated with pain can have a greater impact. There are days when just getting up in the morning is excruciating, and one feels physically and mentally at the end of one's tether. It often helps the person living with chronic pain if there is flexibility in their working hours, and on bad days, the opportunity to do lighter tasks or work a shorter day (what are called 'reasonable adjustments' in the UK). For many people with pain symptoms, part-time work is suitable and, at its best, is an excellent solution. You can negotiate about working part-time with your manager. It's better to reduce your working hours than wear yourself out by working full-time. Today in many countries (with the Nordic countries leading the field), partial sickness allowance makes it possible to continue working part-time while recovering. (The UK equivalent would be a 'phased return to work'.) This speeds up recuperation, and research has shown that the need to take sick leave in the future is reduced by as much as one-fifth. A sickness absence register-based study done by the Social Insurance Institution of Finland, showed that full-time incapacity for work had declined dramatically, by up to two-thirds, at workplaces where partial sickness allowance had been used frequently.

Current knowledge indicates that sick leave in itself hardly ever cures chronic pain. Being at home on sick leave may even prolong and worsen pain symptoms, because at home one's thoughts tend to revolve around pain. Research shows that monitoring one's pain maintains electrical activity in the pain pathways of the central nervous system – in other words, monitoring maintains pain. Worry about the causes of pain, the adequacy of investigations and treatment, and the fear of losing the capacity to work churn around in one's mind at home. The prolongation of symptoms and sick leave raises many questions: who is doing my work? Is anyone doing it? What do my colleagues think? What does my boss intend to do? Why isn't my pain improving? When will I go back to work? Or, can I ever return to work if I my pain gets even worse? How will I manage financially? Why isn't my pain being investigated...?

A long absence from work causes many other problems as well. Many of them are more damaging than the assumed benefits of sick leave: structure and rhythm disappear from life, social contacts are reduced, isolation may set in, occupational self-esteem and sense of competence decline, mood is depressed, lifestyle deteriorates, earnings fall, etc.

It pays to make active efforts to maintain the capacity to work. Studies show that the risk of exclusion from working life begins to increase clearly after six weeks of full-time sick leave. After one year of uninterrupted absence, less than 10 per cent of workers with pain symptoms are able to return to their work. Most of them have lost their capacity to work while passively waiting to heal completely at home.

A Dutch study carried out a comparison of workers with chronic pain, some of whom continued to work while others went on sick leave. The study encompassed more than 200 people living with chronic pain. Five characteristics emerged strongly in the study: those who coped at work had (1) significantly fewer pain-related *fears* and consequently (2) less *avoidance of pain*; (3) they *worried* and were *anxious* because of pain less; and (4) they were *more accepting* of pain. In addition, (5) they had an evidently better sense of *control* of their life.

Everyone should have the right to do suitable work where it's possible to cope with pain. This right shouldn't be taken away by doctors, employers, social security personnel, pension schemes or society's decision-makers. Therefore, it's important that the ability of a person living with pain – someone like you – to work is supported by all possible means and at as early a stage as possible. It's in the best interests of you, yourself, and your family. It's also in your employer's best interests. It benefits the healthcare system, the national economy, and all segments of society. The essential point is that together all parties focus on what you *can* do instead of just getting entangled in what pain prevents you from doing. You, too, can be a person who copes.

My own experience

In my work as a doctor, I too often witness the struggle chronic pain sufferers go through while trying to hold on to their work.

Many pain patients drift out of employment too often and far too early – and too often land on thin air. Exclusion from working life drives people into financial, social and mental/emotional difficulties. It is a great human tragedy that one wouldn't wish on anybody. 'Either-or' thinking – that a person is either healthy or ill, either capable of working or disabled, either on sick leave or working at full speed – still seems to dominate our world view. Attitudes, practices and legislation related to working life generally don't make it easy for people with chronic pain to cope. People in general don't understand well enough that neither chronic pain nor ability to work is an 'all or nothing' condition.

However, not all of the resistance stems from external factors, the work itself, the employer or the legislation. Often, the obstacles to coping at work are grounded in the pain patient's attitudes and expectations or ways of thinking. Many worry about, and are afraid of, how the employer or co-workers will see them and treat them. It is important to understand that many of these work-related fears are produced by a tired mind that's in pain; they don't necessarily reflect reality.

As a doctor, I hear surprisingly often that workers suffering from chronic pain are unwilling to tell their colleagues about their situation, and are especially unwilling to talk to their manager. There are many reasons for this. Pain patients, with their special needs, don't want to stand out from their colleagues because they are afraid of encountering ill-will or lack of understanding. They are perhaps afraid of being seen as a whinger, or perhaps as a scapegoat if things don't proceed satisfactorily. Many feel guilty that others have to do more work. It's often easier to stay away from work completely rather than face these assumed consequences.

In an era of increasing emphasis on productivity, individuals may be afraid of losing their job if they mention being unable to do their work. In the current situation, we may feel we should probably be grateful to have work at all. Some employers are keen to reinforce this impression and stress that only a very limited amount of support is available, if any. Thus workers living with pain are afraid to ask for modifications and special arrangements, especially if something has already been done for their benefit in the past. If special arrangements are made, there is the threat of being seen by colleagues as the boss's pet.

As a pain sufferer, you alone are not responsible for maintaining your capacity to work. The employer has the obligation – and almost always the wish – to support your coping at work. (In the UK you have the support of The Equality Act which includes a duty for the employer to make 'reasonable adjustments'.) I have often heard managers say that they wished they had known about their workers' situation earlier, so that they could have helped in time. It may be difficult to pick up on another's difficulties, especially when pain isn't visible on the surface. It is tragic when, unbeknown to the boss, the worker's condition becomes so bad that he or she eventually goes on long-term sick leave and even becomes incapacitated for work. It may come as a complete surprise to both the manager and co-workers.

We can, of course, also survive from a collapse. As a species, we are survivors and fighters. Over time, we adapt to new situations, including being off work for a long time, and having no regular daily pattern, or social group, to money being scarce and everyday life being confined within the walls of the home. We can become accustomed to that, too. But at that stage, it's much harder for the employer and/or the occupational healthcare service to help a person return to working life.

It's worth talking to your manager. He/she is the one who really can influence things. Emotional support is important, but that alone isn't enough if nothing concrete is done. Small changes in everyday life will often have great effects. Try to see things from your manager's point of view and consider what obstacles and opportunities he/she might have for adjusting your work. When you tell him/her about your problem, suggest a solution as well.

Many chronic pain sufferers end up changing jobs or

occupations, or just quit if it proves to be difficult to cope with pain in their usual work. Before doing that, however, you should devise a clear pain management plan and try all possible means to ease the situation. Major career-related decisions shouldn't be made for flimsy reasons. If treatments are still underway, or inadequate, or if some diagnostic procedures are planned, it may not necessarily be worth starting to train for a long-term change of occupation. The time for that comes only when the pain is being managed better and the person living with pain still cannot cope at work.

In my consultations unfortunately I often encounter patients who, in the end, have lost their capacity to work owing to what their spouse or an acquaintance has said. The spouse's strong views and beliefs about the causes of pain and its care have perhaps paralysed the patient mentally and in part even physically. I hear things like: 'My husband said I can't go to work there and risk injuring my back any more' or 'My wife was afraid that one day I would wind up in a wheelchair if I continued working, and then we couldn't enjoy healthy retirement years together.' Without realising it, a well-meaning spouse, mother or former colleague may reinforce fears about pain, about getting about with pain, and about going to work. It's known that chronic pain undermines self-esteem, makes life uncertain and increases the longing for approval. In such circumstances, what others say can have a surprisingly large impact on the thoughts and actions of a person living with pain.

Learn to trust yourself and your intuition. No one can judge your capacity to work better than you yourself. Only you know what you can do and the kind of work that you could cope with. Hopefully you have already realised that chronic pain is almost never a sign of danger, and that you need not avoid actively living and doing what you want because of it. Maybe you can see working in a new light now. It doesn't pay for you to wait passively to see what others think up for you. Matters proceed best when you yourself take the initiative. Suggest solutions, get the right information (see Chapter 1), ask questions, and ask for help.

My own capacity for work has been tested from time to time. I recognise myself as a typical pain patient: an over-achiever driven by high internal standards whose own wellbeing is trampled by work. I find it difficult to recognise my own limits. I do things myself rather than delegate. I often get absorbed in my work for long periods because the pull of it is too strong.

Fortunately, I have woken up to my situation. The big step has been to recognise – and admit – when too much is too much. My coping has been facilitated by the fact that my work is meaningful and I've been able to adapt it to suit myself. I've needed sick leave very rarely, but I have needed it sometimes. When working with patients, the threshold to staying away from work is very high. If the doctor is away, the help many patients need with their problems is delayed. What's more, the work piles up because locum doctors are seldom available. I guess that's why many doctors would rather go to work sneezing with a stuffy nose, or operate with a foot in a plaster cast, than stay at home and rest.

The possibility of teleworking/working remotely also helps me: I can do written work such as preparing lectures on a laptop more efficiently while sitting in a backward-tilting TV chair than at my office desk. My back was very grateful when, at the beginning of my employment, my boss arranged for an electric adjustable desk in my office. I bought an ergonomically designed office chair from a flea market myself because, having received the desk, I was ashamed to ask my manager for that as well.

I have made compromises with regard to my own career development. For example, I don't apply for managerial positions even though they interest me. This gives me more time to look after my health.

What you can do

- **Learn to recognise your limits.** Don't let your sense of responsibility or your good nature destroy your health. Pace yourself. Rest at times. Adapt mentally to the idea that your capacity to work isn't what it used to be – but you can still cope. Don't blame yourself for having a bad day; we all have bad days. Don't think so much about what your colleagues, your boss or your spouse think. Trust yourself. You know your own field, and your work skills and expertise won't disappear even if your capacity to work is reduced temporarily.
- **Don't blame yourself** because you have been, or currently are, on sick leave. It's not your fault, especially if no work arrangements have been made and your pain hasn't been got under control comprehensively. On the other hand, repeated absence from work isn't in your best interests. Be aware that your risk of becoming permanently incapacitated for work has increased.
- **Think about your own attitudes** towards your work, the meaningfulness of it, the social atmosphere at your workplace, and the relationship between you and your manager – could they have an impact on your pain and your capacity to work? Strive to realise how much your own worries and fears regarding the worsening of pain or permanent disability prevent you from coping at work or returning to working life.
- Appendix 2 to this book presents suggestions regarding the work arrangements for a person living with pain. Go through the list and evaluate which suggestions have been put in place in your case and what you would like to have arranged. You can suggest changes to your manager and / or colleagues.
- It's in your own best interests that your boss keeps in contact with you during your sick leave. He / she's

interested in your health and looks forward to your return to work. Ask to have a soft landing back on the job – for instance, through temporary modifications in work hours or a work trial.

- Job sharing, unpaid leave or some other sabbatical arrangement can be a way, for a little while, to get out of the rat race of struggling with the daily grind and fatigue. You'll get time to care for yourself.
- If you are on long-term sick leave, consider what small steps you could take so that you could return to work, perhaps a 'phased return to work'. Set concrete goals for yourself.
- Make a list of jobs and tasks: what you would like to do; what you're good at; what you're able to do; and what you'd like to learn. Think creatively. Many have made their hobby into a job for themselves.
- Contact your manager or your company's HR office or occupational healthcare service if you are part of a large organisation or, if necessary, the rehabilitation adviser of your pension fund, social security office, or the employment office, and ask about the return-to-work process. At the same time, you can also ask about occupational rehabilitation and work trials. Your locality may have a social services and rehabilitation professional who would be glad to advise you.
- Having their own business or self-employment has been a good solution for many people living with chronic pain. This can provide additional opportunities to tailor your working hours or the amount of work according to your symptoms. Working at home also allows a more flexible pacing of work and also of rest.
- Familiarise yourself with these resources among others: www.nhs.uk/live-well/healthy-body/ways-to-manage-chronic-pain/#go-to-work-despite-the-pain, and www.hse.gov.uk/msd/backpain/workers/work.htm

Chapter 11

Be open to love and affection

The function and structure of the brain change when a person falls in love. Love can be like a drug that causes addiction. It awakens the brain's reward system to demand more. Sleep and appetite may disappear, suddenly energy abounds, and pain isn't felt anywhere. For some, falling in love is a more effective medication than morphine.

But love can also hurt. The word 'heartache' literally means pain of the heart. There are many songs about heartache, and all of them, in slightly different words, tell of how cruelly one's beloved leaves and thrusts a dagger into one's heart. Though it is just a metaphor, the pain is still real: the heart is constricted, with stabs of chest pain.

The loss of love, betrayal and abandonment arouse painful memories even decades later. Physical pain experienced in the past is forgotten more easily than disappointment in love. Loss of love and sorrow can even kill. Many widows and widowers die of broken heart syndrome – or, more formally, 'stress-induced myocardial damage' – soon after the death of their spouse.

Why a person living with pain should love

Love has many manifestations. There's passionate, comradely, platonic, motherly, fatherly and sisterly love; love for one's neighbours, one's pets, food, or a football team.... From the

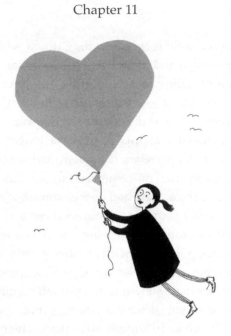

perspective of wellbeing, however, the most important is a healthy and balanced love of oneself. A person who loves him/herself in a good way appreciates, respects, and listens to him/herself. S/he sees the good side of in him/herself and in what s/he does. S/he contemplates what would be good for her/him. S/he looks after and cherishes his/her own body and mind.

Love for another person is also revitalising. Romantic love wonderfully strokes the pleasure centre of the brain and accelerates the production of dopamine. Dopamine is one of the hormones that act as neurotransmitters of the central nervous system – hormones that are central to the pain relief process. Serotonin and endorphins also begin to flow, as does the love hormone oxytocin, produced by touching a loved one and by lovemaking. (More about oxytocin is found in Chapter 4, Don't underestimate the power of touch.)

Falling in love passionately can also be a stressful experience for the body and the mind. The secretion of cortisol increases by 40–50 per cent. The body and the mind are geared for vigilance and action. Psychiatrists recognise the consequences of ardent love particularly well: it is like coming down with mild mania, dementia, obsession and psychosis – all at the same time...

The flame of falling in love doesn't last forever. It changes on average a couple of years after being kindled, or it dies out. When love continues and the couple relationship remains sound, research has shown that this presages a longer, healthier life. Living in a happy couple relationship reduces the need for doctor's visits, and recovery from procedures is quicker. Balanced love also relieves pain and the anxiety and depression associated with pain. When your partner provides encouragement and support, your sense of what you can do is stronger and it's easier to cope with pain. Experiencing intimacy with another person makes it easier to adapt to a temporary worsening of pain symptoms.

Many studies have shown that a person continuing in a bad relationship or living alone experiences more pain and more significant difficulties in coping with pain. Their mood, too, is lower. Naturally it's difficult to say what's the cause and what's the effect.

Why, then, doesn't everyone gravitate towards love to treat their pain? It's not that simple, of course. Sometimes we must go to a lot of trouble, even well beyond our comfort zone, for love. It requires courage. If the reward for the effort isn't as expected, the brain quickly learns that it doesn't pay. Or the other person just doesn't feel right as a partner, no matter how wonderful the individual is otherwise. The cause of this not feeling 'right' may in part be the pain-related disturbed state of the brain's pain regulation and reward system. However, the most important thing is to realise that if you don't love yourself, it may be difficult to accept the love of another person because you don't feel worthy of that love.

What research tells us

Brain research has shown that Cupid's arrow strikes the same areas of the brain as strong analgesics, such as morphine.

Professor Sean Mackey, a pain researcher at the renowned Stanford University, and his team, conducted a study where the volunteer subjects were people, mainly students, in the early stages of falling in love. Like most people who have just fallen in love, they were crazy and silly, euphoric and energetic, and probably a bit trying. Their romantic interest was on their mind constantly, and they had an intense desire to spend all of their time with their beloved.

First, a picture of their beloved was flashed in front of the subjects, and simultaneously the temperature of a thermal sensor placed on their palm was raised with the intention of producing the sensation of pain. At the same time, the subjects' brain function was pictured with a functional magnetic resonance imaging device. Next, they were shown a picture of an attractive person that they knew but with whom there wasn't a romantic emotional bond, and the temperature was raised to exactly the same level.

During the third pain trial, the subjects were asked to do 'neutral distraction' tasks, such as thinking about team sports where a ball isn't used. This was done in order to exclude the possibility that viewing the picture of their beloved would affect the pain only because their attention had been diverted from the pain stimulus. Previous studies have shown that when attention is distracted from the expectation of pain, or the stimulus itself, the pain is not experienced as sharply.

In this particular study, the pain experienced when viewing the picture of their beloved was almost half that experienced when viewing the picture of an attractive acquaintance. Diverting the subjects' attention away from the pain test with the neutral task also relieved the pain, but much greater relief occurred when the subjects viewed their loved one's picture than when their attention was focused elsewhere. The brain imaging showed a lot of activity in the reward centre of the brain. Seeing the loved one's picture produced a reward that effectively countered the pain signals. The more intense the love was (and therefore the greater the reward), the better the pain was averted.

If our love is unrequited, our brain soothes our feelings by producing the same analgesic substances as in physical pain. The more flexible a person's mind is in withstanding such a difficult thing as being turned down, the more the brain produces analgesic substances such as endorphins and the easier it is to get over being rejected. In other words, the brain interprets and treats social pain partly in the same way as physical pain. It is no wonder, then, that heartbreak and physical chest pain feel similar. In fact, ibuprofein and paracetamol ease heartbreak pain, too!

Chronic pain can strain the couple relationship – and strain, in turn, can increase pain. The scientific journal *Pain* published a study on chronic back pain sufferers and their spouses. The study encompassed more than 100 couples, who industriously wrote down their feelings five times a day for two weeks. The more the back pain sufferer experienced criticism and hostility from the spouse, the more intense the back pain was, and the pain did nothing but get worse over the next few hours. The worsening of the pain, in turn, increased the spouse's negative feelings, anger and depression. The spouse's depression further increased the pain experienced by the chronic pain sufferer.

Many people living with chronic pain may be caught up in this sort of vicious circle. It pays to use all possible means to break free of it. Further discussion of this important topic is found in Chapter 6, Talk about your feelings and in Appendix 3 beginning on page 191.

My own experience

In my work as a doctor, I've often encountered pain patients who, in childhood, didn't experience love in a healthy and balanced way. They weren't loved for themselves as ordinary children; instead, they were required to be well-behaved, high achievers, and to hide their negative feelings. Or they were mistreated regardless of how they behaved. In adulthood, this can be reflected in imbalanced personal relationships or lack of social relations. Some may have difficulty relying on others or recognising their own feelings. Others seek the approval they lacked as a child through achievements and sacrifices as an adult.

The suppressed longing for love often manifests itself as wide-ranging, difficult pain conditions, fatigue and depression, an inability to experience sorrow or joy, and sometimes even self-hatred. Such internal stress leads to a prolonged state of agitation in the body that insidiously saps strength. Hyperactivity of the 'accelerating' sympathetic regulation of the autonomic nervous system and the disturbance of 'soothing' parasympathetic regulation are associated with many chronic pain conditions, such as fibromyalgia and irritable bowel syndrome. Many of the tools found in this book specifically target this overly excited state of the nervous system with the aim of calming it and strengthening its functioning.

I have myself travelled a long way on love's bumpy path, stumbling at times but, I am relieved to say, always getting up again. I suppose it isn't easy for anyone to love, but for me the hardest thing has been to learn to love myself, including all of my pain. In the past few years I've worked hard to understand what would actually be good for me, and what I need to do to promote a better life. I've received outside professional help, including cognitive behaviour therapy (CBT), and it has been life-changing for me. The two-year therapy has been a real trip of exploration into myself, and the prize has been many insights and much comfort.

I try to listen to myself. I'm learning to appreciate myself for other things besides achievement and accomplishments. I give myself a pat on the back when I make choices that I know will support my wellbeing in the long run. Such a choice may, for instance, be to leave something undone. I'm learning not to feel guilty when I think of myself and do things for myself.

Along the way, I've also begun to understand what genuine

love for another person is, and how empowering it is to love and feel loved. First of all, I had to realise that I should begin to talk about my feelings. In beneficial love, it is essential to learn to share emotions, including those bad times of unhappiness, frustration and annoyance about not being heard or seen enough. If emotions are just swept under the carpet, buried deep in the soul, they seek another way of manifesting themselves. Pain is one of those ways.

The fact that I've learned to recognise and express my own feelings has given me more health than any exercise or medical treatment.

What you can do

- If you live alone, consider whether there is space in your life for love and a relationship. There are times in life when romantic love is 'right' as well as periods when it isn't, but I believe that the appropriate times are in the majority. When you keep the door open, love creeps in and stays with you. Or it enters with a bang.
- If you are in a relationship, honestly consider whether this relationship is revitalising and beneficial for you, or whether maintaining it drains what little energy you have. If you feel that your present relationship is good, contemplate what particularly makes it so. Weigh this also with respect to your pain. Maintain and strengthen these positive aspects – and remember always to thank your partner.
- If you find that you need a change, take the matter up with your partner in a calm setting when you are both in a relaxed state of mind (neither tired nor when the pain is intense). Plan together how your pain management could be increased through love and affection, and how you could support your partner. It's often helpful for you both

to go together to visit the doctor treating your pain. The right kind of information about chronic pain and other associated symptoms will help your partner to have a more sympathetic and empathetic attitude.

- Chronic pain leads to a lessening of your comfort zone. Be bold and stretch your boundaries. Ask a friend to arrange a date for you, perhaps. The world is full of happy couples who have found each other online. Facebook, Tinder, match.com... Make an interesting profile for yourself, or ask a friend to plan one with you.
- Everyone deserves to be loved. Through therapy, many find love in themselves. Therapy also allows you to begin to recognise and confront your own feelings. Ask your doctor or nurse about the various possibilities for doing this. You can find information on therapy services in your area, for example, here: //www.nhs.uk/conditions/stress-anxiety-depression/free-therapy-or-counselling/
- In addition, learn more about your learned patterns of behaviour ('schemas') that may also be a barrier to love: www.oxforddevelopmentcentre.co.uk/schema-therapy/

Chapter 12

Get a pet

Many pets give their owners sincere love. They don't judge or question, discriminate or criticise. Dogs are a great example of this. When one is seized with gnawing pain and feeling lousy, a dog will gently look deeply into the eyes of its master/mistress and sense what's happening. It can interpret human body language and feelings. It knows when its companion has had a bad day and is not well. It knows that a serious expression and tears are a sign of being unwell. At such times, a dog will lie next to the person who is suffering, refuse to budge and carefully observe what is going on. It is concerned and provides comfort.

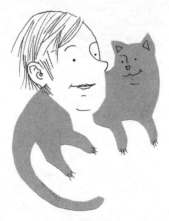

A cat may lift its tail, turn away and disappear, but not because of the person's feelings; it does so because it's a cat and that's how cats behave. Yet a cat, too, knows how to show its love if it wants to. Its affection for a particular person is obvious. A lick of its rough tongue in the morning, a gentle demanding butt of the head when in a soft mood: 'Meow, I'm here, scratch me, cuddle me. And then go quickly to open that food tin.'

Why a person suffering from pain should have a pet

A pet makes a person feel needed and accepted just as s/he is. The closeness of a soft, warm animal calms the mind and body. You can unburden your feelings to your pet, show affection, chat and babble.

Stroking a dog or cat, or even a guinea pig, or a horse, increases the production of oxytocin in the person stroking the animal – and in the animal being stroked, too. Oxytocin is one of the pain-relieving hormones. However, new studies have shown that oxytocin production is stimulated by looking the animal in the eye. Gazing into a dog's gentle eyes raises the oxytocin level in humans dramatically, even tripling it. A dog is a particularly beneficial pet because we can make sustained eye contact more easily with dogs than with other animals. In addition to pain relief, oxytocin improves our ability and desire to get together with other people. A pet helps us make friends, and it's well known that social relationships promote health while loneliness increases our experience of pain.

What research tells us

It has been known for hundreds of years that pets promote health. These effects are quite astonishing, given how little they are used in healthcare. Research has shown that many pet owners are in better than average health: their blood pressure and cholesterol levels are lower, and their ability to ward off infections and tolerate stress is better. Anguish and melancholy are relieved faster in the proximity of a pet, and pet owners generally feel more positive. Recovery from a major shock or a heart attack is generally quicker if there is a pet at home that the patient is waiting to see. Many excellent health effects are linked especially with having a dog, but this phenomenon isn't explained merely by the physical activity of dog-walking.

The role of pets in the treatment of pain is still new, and therefore only a handful of studies are available.

Dog therapy

An American pain clinic studied how pain patients coming for treatment reacted to dog therapy. They offered 235 patients coming to the clinic as well as 34 family members or friends, and 26 staff members the opportunity to stroke and pat a dog for 10 to 15 minutes while the patient was waiting for the doctor. The animal was a well-trained therapy dog that knew how to behave well during these meetings and neither jumped around nor chewed at chair legs. The control group consisted of 95 subjects in the waiting room without any contact with a dog. The members of both groups completed a questionnaire before and after the dog therapy/waiting time. So that the therapy dog wouldn't get too stressed by meeting numerous new people, these encounters were restricted to a few hours a day over a two-month period.

The patients who spent time with the dog, regardless of their diagnosis, reported one quarter less pain than those in the control group. Their pain was clearly alleviated even before they had seen the doctor. Fibromyalgia patients reacted to dogs exceptionally well: their pain was alleviated by one third. The effect was the same as that of analgesics, but more varied. Fatigue and stress decreased among all the patients who spent time with the dog, and they felt calmer and more cheerful. The patients in the other group, who waited for the doctor in the waiting room with old magazines to keep them occupied, felt that their fatigue worsened and they got more tense. Spending time with the dog also felt good; almost all of the patients (92 per cent) were 'satisfied' with their visit to the clinic. Interestingly, satisfaction and the experience of pain relief did not depend on whether the patient considered him/herself a dog person or a cat person. The nursing staff also got to enjoy the positive effects of the dog: Their stress levels fell, too. What's more, in their opinion their relationship with the patients became more positive.

According to another American study, the companionship of a pet reduces the need for analgesics. Trained therapeutic dogs visited patients recovering from joint replacement surgery daily for five to 15 minutes. These visits were a remarkable aid, as the patients receiving animal therapy needed 25 to 50 per cent less painkilling medication than patients who didn't have an animal close by while convalescing.

In a randomised controlled trial of 72 patients undergoing knee or hip replacement surgery, patients were offered physiotherapy on the first three days immediately after surgery. Before the first session, patients were divided into two groups: one spent 15 minutes with the hospital therapy dog before each physiotherapy session and the other went straight to the physiotherapist. The patients who received dog therapy experienced less than half the postoperative pain experienced by the control group. Pain management and doctor-patient communication were also considered to have improved. The patients who had been with the dog were also very happy with the hospital; most of them gave their treatment the best possible grade.

Horses and riding therapy

Some pain patients have said they use riding therapy to treat their symptoms. Surprisingly many have started horse riding only after becoming ill and seeking pain management methods that suited them. While on horseback, pain may disappear, spirits lift, self-esteem and self-efficacy be boosted, and a sense of achievement flourish. There may be some passing soreness after the riding lesson, but this pain is not as unpleasant as the usual pain.

I found just one small study dealing with the effects of riding therapy on chronic pain. According to that study, the pain is relieved, but that is only part of the impact on health. Many other positive effects occur, too: the sense of balance, control of movement and muscle control also improve. Muscles, especially the pelvic muscles and the muscles supporting the back, are strengthened and the rider's body awareness is enhanced. This is especially important for people with prolonged pain, as body awareness begins to blur, and control of movement of the painful limb or body part, and of the entire body, deteriorates. When riding, a person learns to express and regulate his/her feelings better, and anxiety and depression are alleviated.

The same effects have been reported in other health-related studies on riding that haven't actually measured pain. However, all these effects are beneficial to people living with pain.

My own experience

Riding is not for me. I fear and respect large horses too much. Cats, in their turn, perplex me, and their unpredictability always keeps me on my toes. I'm not sure I could totally relax in the presence of a cat; subconsciously I would be waiting for it to attack my toes from its hiding place under the bed. Just the thought of that strikes me as unpleasant, especially because, owing to damage to my sciatic nerve, the feeling of sharp claws in my foot makes my cortical electrogram reading bounce. My subconscious, naturally, is feeding me a line; nice housecats don't attack their owners' toes, do they?

A few years ago I read an article in a scientific magazine with the heading, 'Have you got a four-legged therapist?' The article impressed me, and after reading it I was completely convinced of the health benefits of having a pet. The studies referred to in the article were etched indelibly on my mind. According to those studies, the presence of a pet increases the time a family spends together, promotes their wellbeing, and shortens quarrels between spouses. I decided straightaway to get a dog for my family. Together, the children and I contemplated what breed of dog would be suitable for us. Although I secretly would have liked a big dog, perhaps a golden retriever, I was clear-sighted enough to stick with a small breed. A book borrowed from the library was a great help – it described the 10 easiest dog breeds. Our choice was a Tibetan spaniel.

My family has since greatly enjoyed the good nature and companionship of Oliver, our Tibetan spaniel. Caressing him visibly brings joy and wellbeing to me, living with chronic pain, and to my children. Oliver's existence is without doubt one of the pillars supporting my work and ability to function. Because of him, it's essential to take a walk every day, sometimes even for long distances. Tibetan spaniels aren't friends of long walks, at least not our stubborn Oliver. Every now and then he winds up on a longish walk with me, and that's a real struggle of wills. At the start, I usually have to all but pull him behind me. He turns his muzzle towards home and extends his legs to slow the pace. After a while, he understands that it's no use resisting, and he begins to walk nicely.

I've heard stories from colleagues and have also witnessed in my own patients, how a pet can change a person's life. It's great to see how people who've struggled with pain for a long time begin to regain control of their lives with the help of an animal. Life suddenly has new meaning, a new kind of responsibility, and a more regular rhythm – together with a lot of selfless love and affection. It becomes easier for the pet owner to meet new people with similar interests. For people living with pain, these are all things to encourage so that life can be good, not just constant suffering.

I participated in the thesis a friend was writing for a degree in cultural leadership, the topic of which was the effect of cultural activity on chronic pain (more about this in Chapter 17). More than 100 chronic pain patients responded to a questionnaire dealing with things that enhanced coping with daily life. More than half the respondents reported that a pet gave them strength and resilience in everyday life. A pet was one of the things that helped pain sufferers most to cope with daily living, and it was reported to be almost equal in importance as medical treatment.

What you can do

- If you don't already have a pet, consider the positive contribution one could make to your life. At the same time, consider what you would be willing to give up in order to achieve those positive effects. Is your life situation one that would allow you to get a pet? An animal is a tie, but it also gives a lot.
- One way to try out having a pet is to take care of a friend or neighbour's pet, perhaps while they are away. If you don't know a suitable person to approach, try an advertisement on a pet-focused website or Facebook page.
- If your mobility is limited by pain and you decide to get a dog, you should arrange for a dog walker or a temporary care place for your dog in good time, in anticipation of the days when your pain is too bad.
- When choosing a dog, breed is highly important. Consider whether you would be able to keep a dog weighing 10s of kilos in check when it becomes boisterous.
- Many people living with chronic pain have also become very sensitive to noise, so a breed that's prone to barking easily probably isn't the best choice.
- Mild allergy isn't necessarily an obstacle to having a pet; many people manage well by taking anti-allergy medication for their symptoms, if needed. A difficult case of allergy or asthma is another matter. Then it may not pay

to take the risk that your health might deteriorate. There are breeds of dog that are less allergenic (such as poodles and labradoodles) so it might be worth seeing how these affect you before coming to any decision.

- An adult dog (perhaps a rescue dog whose elderly owner had died) might be easier to cope with than a puppy.
- Information about stables near where you live can be found on the internet. Ask about courses for beginners. At the same time, ask social services whether it would be possible to receive disability support for rehabilitative riding therapy.
- Research has shown that simply watching cat videos on YouTube reduces anxiety and is refreshing. And it gets your mind off pain for a little while.
- Learn how to take good care of your pet. Give it healthy food (not leftover bread and cake!), be active and play with it, stroke it and make much of it. Through your pet, learn how to care for yourself too – your pet will need you to be in good health.

Chapter 13

Manage your weight

Eating involves a lot of pleasure-motivated learning and automated ways of thinking and acting. If a person eats a sandwich while watching the evening news and does this often enough evening after evening, the subconscious will link the two activities. Then, just seeing the news will awaken the craving for a sandwich in the brain. And the fridge will start pulling us towards it like a magnet... When eating awakens a passing sense of feeling good, these two things – eating and feeling good – will become closely associated with each other. As a result, we learn that when help is needed to lift our spirits, we should reach for food or a bar of chocolate. Chocolate brings a momentary rush of feeling good by raising the levels of serotonin in the brain.

On the other hand, when our attempts to lose weight have failed often enough, and we have had repeated disappointments with slimming, we learn that there's no point trying any longer since our weight can't be changed. And neither can our pain.

With this in mind, it's important that healthcare practitioners look at pain sufferers' weight management from a broad perspective, and without arousing feelings of guilt during healthcare visits. Good weight management undeniably has a positive impact on health, including relieving chronic pain. However, the role of excess weight in the context of pain should be kept in proportion. Although it is known that being overweight increases the risk for various types of pain, and that pain increases the risk of weight gain, being overweight alone can seldom be blamed for pain, or pain for excess weight. It may even be that pain and being overweight have common causal factors: both can be the *result*, for example, of heredity and gene function. Research has found that many overweight people are more sensitive to pain than people of normal weight, and for this reason they may be more prone to developing chronic pain.

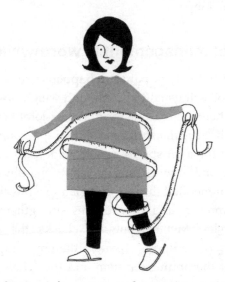

Prolonged insomnia, stress or depression can also be factors underlying chronic pain. They can predispose a person both to being overweight and to suffering from pain by affecting the functioning and structure of the brain and spinal cord. For example, depression is known to interfere with the functioning of the so-called 'descending pain nerve pathways' that suppress pain. There is also some evidence that depression may cause shrinkage of the hippocampus, the brain's memory and learning centre, which plays an important part in, among other things, pacing meal times. When the volume of the hippocampus declines, a person starts eating more often and in greater amounts, resulting in weight gain. Moreover, the significance of low-grade inflammation in the body as a factor underlying pain, being overweight and depression is still not fully understood.

Not all excess weight is lifestyle related. It isn't merely about willpower or self-discipline. A person living with chronic pain may have great difficulties in managing his/her eating in the face of gnawing pain. Eating can be one of the most tempting short-term pain management tools even though the person with chronic pain knows that eating will worsen his/her condition and pain in the long run.

Why weight management is worthwhile

If a person has hip or knee pain and happens to be overweight as well, the doctor will usually recommend weight loss. As dull as that sounds, there are reasons for it. A sore joint benefits from a lighter load. The articular surfaces don't scrape against each other so closely and the joint spaces remain wider. It's easier to cope with daily life and at work, and to follow the physical exercise regimen recommended by a physician or physiotherapist – walking, swimming, and/or exercises strengthening the joint support muscles. Metabolising fat checks the smouldering inflammation of adipose tissue, thereby improving the functioning of the immune system and the whole body. There are other biological benefits, too.

In the case of chronic pain, however, the most beneficial impact of weight management occurs in the mind – the feeling of being in control and slimmer – is best of all. Our self-esteem starts to rise, especially if our weight loss is noticed and praised. Our posture improves and our step becomes lighter. We feel sexier and more energetic. When energy needed for digestion is freed for other uses, we will be less tired. The sense of being more dynamic may increase to such an extent that we need to contemplate where to channel all our energy. What about finally clearing the cupboards or fixing that broken garage door... ?

Our mind and emotions regulate us, whether or not we want them to. In striving to reach a suitable weight, belief that we can do so is crucial. Successful weight management, if anything, gives us the sense that we can influence our own life through our actions and choices. Confidence in ourselves and our own capacities becomes stronger, and self-assurance regarding our own actions increases. It's a boost to discover that the goals we set for ourselves can be achieved, even if they are quite small. All of these factors also support successful pain management.

What research tells us

There are surprisingly few high-quality and large-scale studies that have been able to show that weight loss reduces pain in view of the fact that this connection is considered to be all but self-evident. What's more, the results of the studies that have been done are rather modest: the effect of weight loss on pain relief has been found to be small or at most moderate.

In a Danish study published in 2015, 192 overweight people over 60 years of age with osteoarthritis were distributed into three groups by drawing lots. All of the groups started on a very low energy (about 400 kilocalories (kcal) per day) weight loss programme with the help of meal replacements. Their energy intake was gradually raised to 1200 kcal by adding ordinary food. This strict stage lasted four months, during which time the participants lost an average of 12.8 kg. They were then monitored for a period of one year. During that period, the first group was still offered support for losing weight, the second group was sent for knee-strengthening exercise, and the third group was left to continue as they wished.

As is well known, the most difficult thing about weight management isn't losing weight but maintaining the new, lower weight. Maintaining their weight loss turned out not to be very difficult for the group that received dieting support: a year later, their weight was still 11 kg lower than at the baseline. The second best result was obtained in the group who were left on their own:

a year later, they were still 8 kg lighter. The group that received physical exercise instruction had regained the most weight at the end of the study – their remaining weight loss was around 6 kg, or half of the amount that they had initially lost.

There are many possible reasons why the exercise group had the worst outcome. They were originally the most dissatisfied with their luck in the draw, and not all of them were capable of exercising according to the instructions. The energy-consuming effect of exercise may also have been overestimated. A weight-watcher may think s/he has earned a slightly larger amount of food now that s/he's exercised. What's more, the exertion may make the weight-watcher hungry. Unfortunately, the calories burned in half an hour of sweaty exercise are not great and come back in a few minutes in the form of a slightly larger portion of food or a small chocolate bar. There is also a third possible reason why the exercise group had the worst result: when continuing to exercise felt arduous but weight nevertheless piled back on, their sense of control over their weight, and their belief in their own capabilities and strength, may have weakened as well.

What happened with regard to the test participants' pain symptoms? As far as pain was concerned, this turned out to be a rather typical study. In all of the groups, knee pain was alleviated to the same (small) extent. A year later, they were experiencing about one-tenth less pain – in other words, 90 per cent of the pain was as before. By contrast, many other pains in other parts of the body had increased somewhat, an outcome that probably wasn't caused by slimming, but instead is a relatively commonplace phenomenon associated with chronic pain: the pain changes places.

Other positive effects were observed, however. Quality of life improved by about 20 per cent in the group that maintained the new, lighter weight best. This outcome, in fact, is more significant than the alleviation of pain, as pain and being overweight together worsen the quality of life more than individually. The 'basic pain' of the chronic pain sufferer may not be reduced, but the lighter weight and increased self-assurance make it easier to cope with pain and make life more meaningful.

Prolonged pain is rarely improved *merely* only by losing weight, as also shown by a recent systematic review published in a scientific journal called *Seminars in Arthritis and Rheumatism*. However, weight-loss surgery, after which weight loss may amount to several 10s of kilos, may bring moderate pain relief, though this isn't necessarily reflected in the use of analgesics. An American study focused on almost 12,000 severely obese people who had weight-loss surgery. Some of them were chronic pain patients. Most of the chronic pain patients who used strong analgesics, i.e. opioids, continued to take these medications after their surgery. Among some of them, the need for these medications had actually increased by almost one fifth three years later – even though their weight might have fallen to half of what it had been in the past. The increase in the use of analgesics may indicate that surgery, or indeed dieting, cannot by itself influence the sensitised central nervous system, and therefore chronic pain, in the desired way. The resulting disappointment as the pain persists may surface as an increased need for medication.

For many, eating is a form of subconscious pain management. Studies show that many people living with pain experience pain relief after eating foods rich in fat or sugar. Corresponding changes in the brain have been observed among both chronic pain patients and overweight people: the number of receptors in the brain's endogenous opioid system that produce sensations of pleasure is much lower than the average. It's more difficult for these people to experience pleasure and reward. In consequence, they eat more, and what they eat is more unhealthy. In addition, the nerve impulse messengers, known as neuropeptides, may have a hand here. People living with chronic pain have more neuropeptide Y. These same neuropeptides also convey the sense of hunger to the brain. Thus it may be that people who, for some reason, have an excess of these messengers, experience both pain and hunger more sharply. They are also generally more bad-tempered, as their body aches and their stomach rumbles.

Even short-term daily fluctuations in pain can be seen straightaway in the amount of food consumed: the greater the pain, the more high-kilocalorie food is eaten. Eating sugary treats raises our mood temporarily, and our feelings of being overactive, stressed and in pain improve for a moment. Many overweight people are naturally quite sensitive to the physiological effects of eating. Fat and sugar stimulate the brain to produce its own morphine-like chemicals. In addition, a small sugar rush causes the overactive brain to quieten down for a moment and relieves pain. Unfortunately, the short-term pain relief obtained by eating can lead to a vicious cycle: the weight increases further, the sense of control associated with eating decreases, overall health and fitness weaken, and pain worsens in the long run.

Nowadays, it is better understood how important getting enough sleep is in the management of both pain and weight. Even for healthy people who don't suffer from pain, too little sleep can increase the intake of energy without their even noticing it. In an American study, the sleep of healthy subjects was limited to two thirds of the normal amount. After just a week, their daily energy intake had risen by almost 600 kilocalories even though their energy consumption hadn't increased at all.

My own experience

I don't really believe that healthcare professionals can help their patients to achieve significant weight loss by frightening them or making them feel guilty. Pain sufferers, like everyone else, are equipped with an effective defence system that is quickly activated if the message is wrong or poorly timed, meaning that no message will penetrate through to consciousness. Accepting lifestyle change is each person's own internal process that requires going through a period of reflection and preparation before the individual is motivated to act. Knowledge alone isn't enough. The individual has to realise why a change would be important and beneficial, and why it is worth all the trouble and effort in his/her particular case. For many, that realisation comes only when a colleague or spouse succeeds in managing their weight effectively and then can be seen to flourish as a result of all the effort. The benefits that can be achieved through successful weight control must be made crystal clear to the slimmer. The brain needs to be taught to experience pleasure from things other than food: from an improved appearance, better physical condition, a stronger sense of competence, increased vigour and reduced pain. It pays to strengthen our brain's reward system in all possible situations by praising and encouraging ourselves, and in concrete terms by rewarding ourselves for any success.

In my own weight management, I've experienced the same sort of 'stickiness' as many others. I've begun to think that people with a dysfunctional pain regulation system, such as myself, perhaps can't tolerate a rumbling stomach to the same degree as others. I experience creeping hunger as a very unpleasant sensation. Hunger is too similar to pain, a feeling that I actively want to resist. I know that mild hunger isn't a danger signal for most people in today's world of plenty – any more than is chronic pain (see page xxxi) – and can and should be tolerated. Yet it is 'treated' all too easily by eating. I've made the observation that my slender friends tolerate hunger much better than I do. They think it's just a feeling that will pass soon and doesn't require an immediate reaction. And when they eat, they eat admirably slowly and peacefully, letting their stomach and intestines do their job well. And their brain. They don't wolf down their food as though they were afraid that it will run out too soon. The brain infers that hunger has been satisfied after a certain delay in which time the satiety hormones increase. The production of these hormones begins only about 20 minutes after we start to eat.

I wouldn't want this to sound like an excuse, but the bitter truth is that migraine is a miserable disease for a weight-watcher, especially for a person with an all-or-nothing character. I haven't always had the patience to wait for the results of eating just a little bit less; instead, my slimming programme has been too rigorous. In consequence, my blood sugar has fallen, I've come down with an infernal headache, been bad-tempered and lost my enthusiasm for losing weight very quickly. Fortunately, I've learned from this and can now take a more relaxed approach. In other ways, too, I'm learning to go easier on myself. Weight is just one aspect of pain management, and as I've shown in this chapter, it is not the most important one.

What you can do

- Start by thinking about the importance of eating and weight for your own wellbeing and experience of pain. Get a concrete picture in your mind of all the benefits successful weight management can bring to your life.
- Set an overall goal for yourself. Make it realistic and divide it into intermediate goals. If you want to lose 15 kilos, an intermediate goal might be four kilos. Reward yourself, for instance with new clothes. Glow with a sense of wellbeing. Enjoy being slimmer. Take pleasure in being able to control what you do.
- Write your goal down on paper and be committed to it. When your initial enthusiasm begins to fade after a couple of weeks, stop and imagine yourself as you would like to be when you have achieved your goal. That will give you new strength. Take small steps and don't try to change everything all at once.
- Think positively. Don't grieve for the foods you have to cut down on. An absolute refusal to eat certain foods isn't

necessarily the best solution, as it can further increase the craving for a particular food. See an opportunity in new options, use creativity, and be brave.

- Be selfish about your goal.
- If you feel like it, share your goal about slimming with your friends and loved ones. Ask your partner and/or family to be flexible and support you in your goal. Ask them for positive feedback and encouragement.
- Be honest with yourself. Get on the scales so that you know your current weight. When you lose weight, continue to weigh yourself. Once a week is fine.
- Make the table you will eat at look attractive and inviting; enjoy your food with all your senses; eat slowly, chewing properly; to stop yourself eating too much, keep pots and pans on the cooker, don't place them in front of you on the dining table.
- As dull as this may seem, the truth is that dieters should avoid alcohol. An average pint of British lager contains 180 calories, the equivalent of a slice of pizza according to Drinkaware UK or 15 lumps of sugar at 12 calories each.
- Social support helps many dieters.
- Join a weight management group (such as Slimmers' World or Weight Watchers, which can be found online) or invest in a personal trainer.

Chapter 14

Give up smoking

When pain has begun to control our life, we try to ease it by any possible means. For some, one such means is tobacco smoking. Smokers say they can relax with a cigarette and a cup of coffee. Nicotine clings to the nicotine receptors of the central nervous system with intense force, and the pleasure centre of the brain begins pumping dopamine into the bloodstream. As a result, a feeling of pleasure spreads through the body and pain is mercifully relieved – at least for a moment.

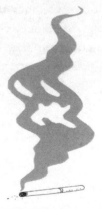

Smokers feel that they get other rewards as well: a cigarette break during an intense workday gives the sore body and tired mind the chance to have a brief moment of relaxation. Among fellow smokers one usually hears the day's best and raciest stories, and laughter makes one forget any pain. Smoking also involves a sense of community: it means that something in common is shared with others at the workplace.

The worst-case scenarios associated with smoking (such as cancer and chronic lung disease) may seem meaningless when pain has already consumed the joy of living and, at its worst, even cost one the ability to work or move around. In such a situation, one clings to small sources of pleasure even if they are known to be unhealthy. Many pain sufferers may think that analgesics are still worse poison than tobacco. Or that pain has just used up so much of their strength that the idea of quitting seems impossible.

Why a person living with pain should stop smoking

Smoking has a wide range of biological effects that are known to increase the risk that pain symptoms will become chronic, and also get worse. These risks include, among others, compromised circulation, stronger inflammatory reactions, disruption of intervertebral disc metabolism, increased tendon brittleness, and even increased gene-level mutations. The body and brain of smokers age more rapidly than normal. The use of opioids is more common among smokers because they are more vulnerable to becoming addicted to them. According to brain research, smoking reinforces activity especially in areas of the brain that process addiction, motivation and learning. These same areas also play a key role in pain becoming chronic.

The good news is that once a person has stopped smoking, nature corrects a large share of the cell-level damage. In practice, however, this knowledge is seldom enough to motivate us to give up a physiologically highly addicting habit that has a strong direct effect on the brain's reward system. I believe that giving up smoking in itself is a more meaningful reward for a person living with pain, as it strengthens their sense of control and achievement. You will find that when you can control your cravings better, you will also be able to control many other things: your thoughts and notions about yourself; the course of your life; your pain. With regard to giving up smoking, it probably isn't an exaggeration to say that if you're able to control something so chemically addictive, you can do anything!

What research tells us

Stopping smoking is a potentially effective pain management tool in the long run. One of the largest studies published so far is based on patient data held by the University of Rochester Medical Center in New York, which relates to over 5300 Americans. They all had back pain, either local lower back pain or sciatic pain radiating to the lower limb, and had wound up in hospital care because of their back pain. Some of them underwent back surgery during the follow-up period, but most of them received so-called conservative treatment, such as physiotherapy, analgesics, exercise instruction and cortisone or anaesthetic injections. All were asked about their smoking status and all of the smokers were advised to stop.

These patients were monitored for an average of eight months. At both the beginning and end of the follow-up, there was less back pain among those who had never smoked or who had stopped smoking before the study began. Pain was more common among the smokers. What's more, the pain they experienced was stronger on all indicators of the visual analogue scale that was used to measure pain: the strength of pain at the time of questioning and during the previous week, and the worst pain experienced.

During follow-up, back pain was relieved among both the non-smokers and those who had stopped smoking. The pain was relieved especially among those who had stopped smoking during the study. What about those who had continued smoking? Their pain was hardly alleviated at all during the entire follow-up period. That's a shame, because the evidence shows that also one's mood picks up when one stops smoking.

Chronic pain is often associated with anxiety and depression, and people who are anxious and depressed smoke more than others. Scientific evidence on the impact of giving up smoking on these symptoms is surprisingly strong.

A large-scale meta-analytical study collating the results of 26 individual, good-quality follow-up studies was published in the prestigious *British Medical Journal* in 2014. The carefully collected and re-analysed data indicated that stopping smoking clearly reduces the symptoms of depression and anxiety, and the experience of stress. Quitting also promoted being in a good mood, and significantly improved quality of life. Most astonishingly, the effects of putting out that last cigarette on mood were even stronger than, or at least as strong as, the effects of antidepressants. Cost-effective treatment, so to speak.

My own experience

To my disgrace, I admit to having smoked for almost 30 years. A few cigarettes a day, often none at all; but when I was younger, a whole pack might go during an evening at the pub. Not even the post mortems of lung cancer patients that were part of my medical studies banished smoking from my life. Indeed, after those I probably puffed away twice as much, to soothe my nerves.

Fortunately, nine years ago I found the resolve to stop. Even then, it happened only after I'd had quite a shock. Namely, I was among those unlucky enough to go down with swine flu. One day my temperature shot up to 40°C, and my lungs were horribly clogged. I ended up in a hospital emergency room and was put on an oxygen respirator. It was a ghastly experience, but luckily I pulled through. And luckily I was frightened enough to stop smoking. I decided that I would start protecting my lungs. Giving up smoking has had no effect on my back pain symptoms, but it has meant fewer headaches and migraine attacks.

What you can do

- Think about the importance of smoking to you. How does smoking make you feel? Does it act as a means of stress management? Or as a momentary numbing of your pain? Are there alternative ways to relieve stress or relax described in this book that could help you?
- Talk with friends and/or colleagues who have stopped smoking. How did they do it? What positive effects have they experienced once they quit? What have they gained in the place of their beloved cigarettes? How have they managed to stay clear of smoking?
- Also ask your doctor about the experiences of other patients once they've been able to stop smoking. Ask what kinds of positive effects, both physically and mentally, can be expected after quitting.
- Yoga, mindfulness, hypnosis, acupuncture and/or medical treatment can also help you to give up smoking. Ask your doctor or nurse about them, or find out more here: www. nhs.uk/smokefree/help-and-advice/ecigarettes-and-hypnotherapy
- If you're a heavy smoker and take medication both for pain and for depression, calculate how much money you could save in a year if you were to stop smoking. Do different calculations including one where you wouldn't spend a penny on cigarettes, another where you wouldn't need antidepressants, and another where the need for analgesics would be cut in half.
- Smoking and opioids can reinforce each other so that dependence on each of them only deepens. Consider which

of them would be easier to give up first. Do it in small steps, but purposefully. Consider which of the people in your close circle could support you during this change, and ask her/him for help.
- Good information is available on these websites:
  www.nhs.uk/smokefree
  www.quit.org.uk/about/

Chapter 15

Try yoga

Do you check your emails/social media many times an hour? Do you stop reading a newspaper to look at Facebook updates? Do you pour coffee from the pot before it's finished dripping through the filter? So do I (sigh).

We live at an accelerating pace. People are more short-tempered. The concept of time is changing. What we used to accomplish in a week should now be done in a day. Careers have been disrupted by outsourcing and freelancing. Demands for efficiency are increasing. Even being a parent all but requires the competence of a logistics manager (another sigh).

It's no wonder that people long for ways to stop and find calm. Yoga is an excellent tool for this because it combines physicality and spirituality, exercise and meditation, in a versatile manner. The body can exert a strong influence on the mind, and vice versa.

In a study conducted in the US, one in 10 people reported doing yoga. In Europe, too, yoga's popularity has been rising so sharply that it has clearly come to stay. People do yoga at their workplaces, in groups in parks, in old-age homes where residents do chair yoga; children in day-care have fairytale yoga. Yoga classes can also be attended at home virtually, through online contact with the instructor and the rest of the group.

This is good news! The yoga boom is certainly influenced by people's increased awareness of, and interest in, their own

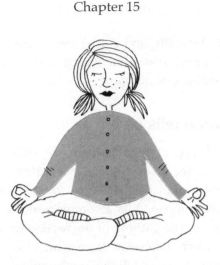

wellbeing and health. The connection between the body and the mind is understood better (thanks, for instance, to brain research). Conventional Western medicine hasn't been able to meet people's need for holistic therapies. Attention has turned towards safe and evidence-based complementary therapies, especially when dealing with chronic pain problems, and their use appears to be increasing.

Why a person living with pain should try yoga

Yoga is an excellent combination of training for the body and for the mind. It can help to facilitate pain management, improve mobility, raise spirits and relieve anxiety. It can also dispel the fatigue associated with chronic pain. Many kinds of yoga are available, and in many places. Starting to do yoga doesn't require more than an open mind, flexible clothes, a firm surface or mat and instruction.

In principle, yoga is a safe form of exercise, but it may not be suitable for everyone suffering from chronic illnesses. For instance, if you have been diagnosed with a significant spinal disc herniation that gives rise to symptoms, it is advisable to consult the doctor treating you before you sign up for a yoga class. It's a good idea to start with a form of yoga that is the lightest physically, and it isn't necessary to do all of the movements. If a particular movement doesn't feel suitable, skip it and do something else instead.

What research tells us

Out of all the effects of yoga on pain, the effect on back pain has been studied the most. In 2013, according to a systematic literature review published in the *Clinical Journal of Pain*, yoga can be recommended as a complementary treatment for chronic back pain. The authors of the review went through the five largest research databases, from which they selected only the studies with the most reliable methodology. The selection criterion was strict: the study design had to be a randomised comparison. Randomisation means in practice that the test subjects may not choose their treatment mode, but that they are assigned to different groups by lot. The review encompassed about one thousand adults with chronic back pain who had consulted healthcare professionals. According to the authors, there was strong scientific evidence for the short-term effects of yoga and moderate evidence for its long-term benefits. Then in 2017, a highly respected Cochrane Systematic Review concluded, after reviewing 12 studies, that yoga results in small to moderate improvements in back-related function and may also be slightly more effective for pain compared with not exercising at all. Considering that no treatment for chronic low back pain is superior and none has been shown to lead to considerable improvements as such, the result from the Cochrane Review can be considered significant.

Migraine headache is one of the worst pains anyone can experience. At its most severe, a migraine attack is completely disabling – it can cause functional incapacity for hours or even days. More than half of those with migraine experience attacks at least once a month; and one in 10 have an attack weekly. It is therefore gratifying to read studies indicating that regular yoga reduces the number of migraine attacks and their intensity. Several recent systematic reviews, one being published in the prestigious *British Medical Journal* in 2017, have concluded that yoga has a positive effect on migraine and headache. Yoga doesn't have to be done for hours a day to achieve these results; half an hour is enough. Regularity is more important.

The effects of yoga aren't limited to alleviating back pain or headache. Women with pelvic pain benefit from yoga, as is shown by a recent systematic review. The pain and weak grip associated with carpal tunnel syndrome have also been reduced by yoga exercises, as have osteoarthritic pains in the small joints of the hands and knees, fibromyalgic pain and post-menopausal pain and fatigue. People with chronic fatigue syndrome also seem to benefit from yoga. According to some studies, the impact of meditation and yoga on pain is even greater than the impact of painkillers.

These results are also supported by the latest studies on pain, based on brain imaging. The studies have made it possible to demonstrate objectively that yoga alters the functioning of pain pathways in the cerebral cortex. The same effect has also been observed for meditation. In addition, practising yoga has the opposite effect of chronic pain on the brain. It seems to prevent the reduction of, or even increase the amount of, grey matter in the brain. Decreased grey matter has been linked to memory impairment, emotional problems and reduced cognitive functioning. Long-term yoga practitioners and meditators are better able to establish a durable state of mental silence. That silence is not easily disturbed by chronic pain.

My own experience

During the writing of this book, I finally began to do yoga. I had been aware of its health effects for a long time, and had directed many of my patients to take it up. For some reason, the threshold to seeking out yoga classes for myself had nevertheless been high. Now that I've overcome that, the experience of yoga has been so rewarding that I intend to continue. The feeling I get after a lesson is simultaneously both energised and comfortably soft and relaxed – as if I had flown from Finland to Australia and back in economy class with my knees jack-knifed and could finally stretch once the plane had landed. What a blissful feeling!

What you can do

- There are many different kinds of yoga groups for different needs: yoga for men, hot yoga, mother and baby yoga...
- Hatha yoga can mean very many different things. Gentle Hatha yoga usually suits everyone. Yin yoga involves very slow stretching. Astanga is physically more demanding, not perhaps something for a beginner.
- Open colleges, sports halls, outdoor exercise organisers and many others offer yoga classes; look online or in your local newspaper. Try it. Borrow a yoga mat from a friend to see how you get on, then buy your own. Normally, the content of any yoga course is explained upon enrolment. Start from the lightest alternative and, if you wish, proceed gradually to more demanding types.
- I recommend sometimes trying a well-known yoga instructor's lessons. A luminary yogi can bring tangible charisma and energising spark.
- You can also spread your own yoga mat on your living room floor. Put on flexible clothes, open your laptop and find a YouTube video with yoga instruction for beginners, for example on NHS's website:www.nhs.uk/conditions/nhs-fitness-studio/yoga-with-lj/?tabname=pilates-and-yoga. There are also online yoga services where the instructor

gives yoga lessons remotely.
- Go to yoga classes with a friend or your partner, or do yoga together at home. A yoga holiday in a wellness centre, or even in a holiday resort, will perk up everyday life.

Chapter 16

Try acupuncture

If you've never tried acupuncture, you may perhaps consider it a mystical type of alternative medicine. Actually, it's a form of treatment used by many quite down-to-earth people. Many doctors and physiotherapists have learned to give acupuncture even though they wouldn't otherwise be interested in complementary treatment methods. They have just found that acupuncture works.

The effects of acupuncture have been tested for almost 4000 years. Originally developed in China, it gained a strong foothold in Western medicine decades ago. Today, it has an established position in many countries' Current Care Guidelines as a useful method for treating various pain states.

In acupuncture treatments, a trained healthcare professional inserts very fine needles into the skin at designated acupuncture points, and also into the muscles or the fascia surrounding these, where sensitive or sore areas – so-called trigger points – are felt. Trigger points are knots that move under the fingers when kneaded and which may cause the patient to twitch and yelp.

The tip of the acupuncture needle, which is nearly as thin as a hair, pierces the skin to a depth of just a few millimetres. Most people don't feel anything much when the needle is put in. To take effect, the needles remain in place for 10 to 40 minutes. According to traditional Chinese thinking, most acupuncture points lie on invisible channels, called meridians, through which blood and energy flow. These points are stuck with acupuncture needles in an effort to influence the energy that flows through the meridians. If a channel is blocked, the blockage is felt as pain or some other symptom. The goal of inserting pins into the trigger points of muscles is to relax cramps and relieve pain.

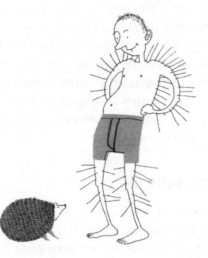

Why a person living with pain should try acupuncture

To improve pain management, acupuncture is definitely a tool worth trying. In skilled hands, it is a safe treatment method, and it is now available in many places providing care, at least in larger towns and cities. Four to eight treatments are usually enough to provide pain relief and the effect is shown to remain for up to 12 months, according to a systematic review published in the highly respected journal *Pain* in 2017. Some people treat their migraines by having a series of four or five treatments once or twice a year, which keeps their symptoms at bay. In addition to pain, acupuncture can be used to treat many other complaints, such as insomnia, anxiety, sweating and intestinal ailments.

Many chronic pain sufferers have been helped by acupuncture. It has very few side-effects, although some people may have a mild headache after the first treatment, especially if they have been treated for complaints of the neck and shoulder region. It is said that mild headache would be due to healing of the circulatory system, and to the fact that waste-products start to leave muscles.

Many people say that they've had a passing feeling of pleasant euphoria after treatment. They feel soft and light. One of my patients has said that acupuncture had the same relaxing impact as a glass of wine. People usually sleep well the night after a treatment. For many, relief from muscle tension begins during treatment itself, with a feeling of warmth in the muscles and a slight tingling. The pain-relieving effect usually begins only after the second treatment.

What research tells us

Acupuncture has been in use by Western conventional medicine for so long that a good deal of research data has accumulated to support it. Dozens of meta-analyses have combined data from individual studies. One of the largest of these includes a meta-analytical study, published in the *Journal of Pain* in 2018 covering 20,827 patients from 39 trials. The authors of the review went back to the original research material and made additional analyses from the data. Their final conclusion was that acupuncture is effective for the treatment of chronic musculoskeletal, headache and osteoarthritis pain. In addition, as mentioned above, treatment effects of acupuncture persist over time and cannot be explained solely in terms of placebo effects.

In another review, acupuncture appeared to be even more effective than conventional pain management, which in practice means taking analgesic medications.

According to another published meta-analytical review, acupuncture can raise the pain threshold both of healthy people and of people living with chronic pain. More than 80 per cent of the almost 100 studies selected for the review showed increased tolerance of pressure following acupuncture (pressing pain points no longer felt as painful). Over 60 per cent of the studies indicated that treatment with acupuncture helped people to tolerate pain caused by cold or heat.

Acupuncture most likely affects pain through multiple mechanisms. The energy flow through meridians is probably the 'non-scientific' explanation. Scientifically, it has been possible to verify many ways in which acupuncture relieves pain. Brain research has also been helpful in this. Several studies using functional magnetic resonance imaging (fMRI) of the brain have been able to demonstrate how acupuncture modifies the functioning of the brain regions involved in handling pain (even though the needles are inserted into the painful back or neck and not the brain...). At the same time, the functioning of the nerve pathways that dampen pain is intensified, and the signal rising from the painful area to the brain along the nerve pathways is weakened by treatment with acupuncture.

In addition, acupuncture acts in the same way as touch in relieving pain: irritating acupuncture points with a needle closes the 'gate' to pain signals leaving the painful area (more about this in Chapter 4). Acupuncture also stimulates the brain to produce morphine-like chemicals. Euphoria is a consequence of acceleration in the production of endorphins, the feel-good hormones. Also, the levels of neurotransmitters involved in the treatment of depression, such as noradrenaline and serotonin, increase after treatment with acupuncture. At the same time, the overactivity of the sympathetic nervous system often associated with chronic pain is reduced.

My own experience

I administer acupuncture to my patients, and I use it to treat my own pain. I personally benefit from it, and I especially enjoy the immediate euphoric feeling that it gives. Acupuncture also saved my holiday trip a few years ago. At the time I spent far too much time sitting – while writing the original version of this book – and my sciatic pain flared up. I was able to walk only a short distance before the pain became intolerable. I was leaving soon for Madrid with my children, and I began to feel desperate: how would I be able to get around there, in addition to coping with the long flight? I was even considering cancelling the trip, which would be completely exceptional for me. That indicates how strong my pain was.

Fortunately, I managed to get myself to a competent physiotherapist, and I asked for acupuncture. Two treatments with four days between – and the relief was instantaneous. Naturally I was so enthused by my pain-free state that I made a new personal walking record in Madrid: one evening I noticed that, according to the pedometre on my smart watch, I had walked 17,000 steps that day! The sciatic nerve made its unhappiness known back at the hotel room in the evening, but I didn't really notice the pain during the day.

I'm repeatedly surprised at how often chronic pain patients haven't even tried acupuncture. They may have gone through a number of operations and taken lots of medications. Their ability to work may be in question or already have been lost. Yet such a simple and, at its best, highly effective treatment isn't even suggested! Perhaps acupuncture hasn't been available adequately, or doctors haven't known to recommend it.

Nor does fear of needles prevent treatment with acupunture. I've treated many patients who shuddered at the thought of injections and needles, but once they tried it, found that acupuncture didn't bother them. Nowadays in my acupuncture treatments, to enhance the effect, I always simultaneously use a mental image exercise called 'Visualise your soul's landscape' (see Chapter 5, page 42) or I play a 10-minute mindfulness video from YouTube (called 'Guided Mindfulness Meditation for Coping with Chronic Pain').

What you can do

- Many doctors working at health centres and in private practice give acupuncture, so it pays to enquire about this. In the last few years, many physiotherapists have also studied acupuncture and now use it actively. More information about acupuncture can be found from the NHS's website: www.nhs.uk/conditions/acupuncture/
- A good selection of practitioners can be found on the websites of the The British Acupuncture Council (www.acupuncture.org.uk) and the Acupuncture Society in the UK (www.acupuncturesociety.org.uk/find-a-practitioner)
- A list of acupuncture providers with knowledge of traditional Chinese medicine can be found online here: www.atcm.co.uk/find-a-practitioner
- If you are completely unfamiliar with acupuncture, you can watch one of the many YouTube videos which provide an introduction to the topic, for example from the National Center for Complementary and Integrative Health US, link here: www.youtube.com/watch?v=JnKPNw9K2Ng.

Chapter 17

Be creative

Creativity is an integral part of humanity. Many of us are constantly creating something new, designing our garden, restoring old flea market finds, writing journals or compiling songlists in Spotify, which we share on social media. We do it for our own pleasure or for the general good, at the request of other people, or sometimes in spite of what others say. The best moments in the creative process, when we are in a 'state of flow', occur when a mini-nirvana sweeps us along with it. All thoughts centre on what's being done, and the sense of time marvellously disappears. Then we don't remember being poor or ill or in pain.

Living with chronic pain tests creativity. Our main goal becomes trying to cope with everyday life. That is a challenge that can block even the most creative personality and induce the most flexible mind to stick rigidly to unbending thought patterns and daily routines. A person who mentally struggles to keep their head above water (and does it for years and years) doesn't think when paddling on the beach: 'That lifebuoy would be more cheerful if painted yellow.'

With regard to pain management, however, creative thinking is that lifebuoy. Creativity is what provides life support during the difficult moments of everyday life. What's more, a flexible mind is able to see and do things differently. A creative person is curious, daring to seek new solutions and try them out courageously and spontaneously. By experimenting, a person adjusts to new situations and reinforces his/her belief in him/herself and his/her doings. Through successes, the individual starts to see him/herself in a more positive light.

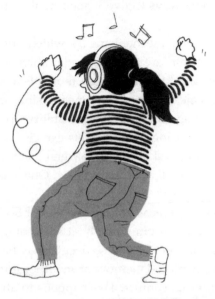

Creative thinking and a flexible mind are worth maintaining and training. Great tools for this are culture and the arts – both appreciating them and taking part oneself. 'Culture and the arts' may sound unnecessarily grand – one's own enthusiastic hobby crafts, DIY, writing poems, shaping bits of wood or weaving rugs, may not seem all that cultural or artistic. That, however, is exactly what they are. They involve nothing less than making something oneself, or enjoying the creations of others.

Why a person living with pain should give free rein to their creative side

Engaging in cultural activities prolongs life more than losing weight, say many scientists after studying the relationship between culture and health. Adding a few years of struggling with pain to one's life isn't the best incentive for someone living with chronic pain to take an interest in culture. I reckon they will be more interested in the knowledge that culture and the arts can help one find new ways to live a good-quality, meaningful life despite pain.

There are several mechanisms by which cultural activities alleviate pain. These are much broader than just 'distracting one's attention' and 'diverting one's thoughts away from pain'. The arts can be a means for overcoming invisible or even concrete obstacles that maintain pain and inability to function. For example, when dancing one also gets exercise, almost without noticing. Mindfulness skills develop when one focuses on crafts, arranging flowers or listening to music. One's sense of power and control increases.

I feel sure you can recall at least one film or book that has had a great impact on you emotionally at some stage in your life. The reason why it touched you so deeply may have been that it triggered a deeply buried memory of an important event in your life, or some internal conflict. This happens to all of us since all of us have suppressed feelings that are difficult to deal with, or even to recognise.

One manifestation of suppressed emotions is chronic pain (there is more about this in Chapter 6, Talk about your feelings). Grief, anger and/or bitterness can be channelled into creative activity or music (performance or appreciation) and given more positive expression, thereby relieving the pain. The experience of pain can also be transferred concretely – for instance, to a drawing or clay model you create – thus giving shape to pain. Culture and art help us to recognise our own strengths and resources that may have been belittled in the past, or considered self-evident. Through art, we can also have a moment as someone else, experiencing the emotions of another person and mirroring them onto our own.

What research tells us

Let's start with music, the art form for which there is the most scientific evidence in the treatment of both acute and chronic pain. This evidence is really convincing. Listening to one's favourite music on a daily basis has been shown to reduce chronic pain by as much as 20–25 per cent. This is quite a good result in view of the fact that analgesics, on average, reduce pain by around 30 per cent. What equally effective means is there available as easily and cheaply – or even free of charge – and almost without side-effects?

Listening to pleasurable music during surgery, even when under anaesthesia, relieves pain, cuts the need for analgesics and reduces anxiety, as shown by a meta-analysis based on research data from over 70 studies and published in *The Lancet*, one of the most prestigious scientific journals. Music is also helpful after surgery. For a Finnish doctoral dissertation, patients who had undergone abdominal surgery listened to music in hospital on the days following their operation. Many of these postoperative patients were surprised at how much the music helped their recovery. Not only did the pain seem milder and less unpleasant, but listening to music also helped them to fall asleep and to relax. Nor did lying in a hospital bed seem as boring when listening now and then to hard rock or pop songs (or any favourite music) through a headset.

Music has also been shown to relieve pain associated with other procedures. The dentist's drill doesn't hurt as much when the patient listens to music at the same time. It's easier to cope with chronic pain, such as fibromyalgia, with the help of music. Movement is eased. Music provides relief even for the pain of cancer and reduces the need for strong analgesics.

Music seems to intensify the functioning of our pain pathways, or so-called 'descending pathways', that block pain signals. The brain's reward system is activated, and the production of good hormones is accelerated. The effects can be seen in brain images quite broadly – not only in the brain but also in the brainstem and even the spinal cord. It's been said that great music can send a cold shiver down the spine...

Music also helps to create positive mental images that displace negative self-perceptions and feelings about the world, at least for a while. It can quickly and easily raise mood, which in turn relieves pain. Music is like a time machine: it can transport a person back in time. Songs act as anchors helping people to attach events and states of emotion to the timeline of their life, and to recognise causal connections between major life changes and the onset or worsening of pain symptoms.

One good side of music as a pain-management tool is the fact we usually have the strength to listen to music, no matter how depressed and paralysed we are by pain. There is also positive scientific evidence regarding music as a complementary form of treatment for depression. It's a good idea to combine listening to music with relaxation exercises, thereby teaching the brain to link the two activities: when repeated often enough, simply listening to music will relax both the mind and the body. Needless tension is eased; so, too, is pain.

Dancing is a good way to combine the positive effects of music and exercise. In particular, dancing relaxes muscle tension and relieves stress and depression, improves sleep at night and, above all, increases our ability to manage chronic pain. According to a scientific review published in 2019, dance practice produces significant positive changes in the structure and function of the brain.

Colour, shape and light have a healing effect, as was noted by the British nurse Florence Nightingale, a model and pioneer of modern nursing, already in 1860. She also pointed out that the effect must be physical and physiological, not just mental. Research has shown that an aesthetically pleasing environment does in fact increase wellbeing. The pain threshold and pain tolerance even of healthy individuals are raised merely by showing them beautiful pictures. It seems this was understood better in the past, when many former sanatoria were located in places of great natural beauty, with arched windows and fountains beautifying the hospital environment. Fortunately, art has again been introduced into many new hospitals. Also, decorating and making the home attractive are positive activities for many people living with chronic pain even though they don't always recognise that such activities are useful for pain management.

Studies, mainly among people with fibromyalgia, have shown that expressing oneself by writing can alleviate pain and ease accompanying symptoms. According to a review by the distinguished Cochrane group, women who suffer from chronic pain in the pelvic region (which, by the way, is a common complaint) benefited from therapeutic writing, which brought about significant pain relief. The effects, however, were found not to last very long, so it pays to make writing a regular habit.

Various art therapies have shown to alleviate pain symptoms even among cancer patients. Professional art therapists to instruct people in making art are useful but not always necessary to achieve the benefits of creating art. In a suitable and encouraging environment, works of art spring from the individual on their own.

Peer group support can help to maintain creative self-expression. In one study, American women with a chronic disease (that almost always involved pain) and living in small towns or in the countryside, were followed-up for a three-month period. They were invited to join an online peer support group where they received health information and were also able to discuss their health status. The important part of the intervention was that group members were also allowed to exchange practical instructions and advice on creative hobbies, such as handicrafts.

The results were positive. Every third participant, on her own initiative, talked about the importance of creative activity as a pain management method. Messages expressed how painting with watercolours led to a state of flow, at the same time making painful finger joints more supple. Drawing made some of the women forget their negative thoughts related to illness. Crocheting was mentioned as a meditation-like activity. Doing crafts, such as making greetings cards for family and close friends, reduced their obsessing about how bad they felt and forced them, in a good way, to think of others and to be social. A positive sense of self was reinforced. Creative activity didn't bring any negative emotions to the surface, or at least such feelings weren't mentioned in the group.

In a recent British study among 2600 older adults, participating in cultural activities, such as going to concerts, the theatre or the opera, or visiting museums, art galleries and exhibitions, significantly reduced the risk of developing chronic pain. The risk reduction was considerable – 25 per cent – and is directly comparable to the risk reduction related to vigorous physical activity. This study is another good example of the psychological benefits that come from social engagement and having positive cultural experiences. Feeling good, or being moved by an impressive piece of art, is, however, not just a feeling. It is a biological event which produces measurable physiological reactions and, consequently, health benefits. Its effects are powerful in healing.

My own experience

When living with chronic pain, it's especially important to cherish things in life that make you feel good. Dabbling in activities I enjoy is one of these things for me. Interior decoration, refurbishing old furniture, crafts, writing... Fulfillng myself and creating something new are perhaps my most important ways of managing my pain. I don't let the pain control me, because life still holds so many fun things to do.

Doing what I enjoy *in moderate doses* is a personal challenge. Enthusiasm and flow easily carry me away, and I don't remember to take breaks. In the last few years, I've had less strength for decorating and DIY before, but nowadays I enjoy music all the more. I've made it into a real pain management method for myself.

I'm not from a musical family, I can't play an instrument or sing very well. Yet it would be difficult to imagine my life without music. One day while writing this book, I was thinking about what music means to me. I realised that, for me, it has always worked as a channel for expressing my feelings. I wasn't very good at recognising my emotions or expressing them in the past, yet I could compile a list of my all-time top 20 power songs in an instant. All of the songs on the list interpreted precisely the emotional states I had experienced at certain stages of my life.

I've also realised that I can alter my feelings with the help of music. This is beneficial when living with pain, which can be quite an emotional roller-coaster. One has to go to work in the morning, no matter how much pain one has or how tired or annoyed one may be. I increase my pain tolerance and raise my spirits on my way to work by blasting Metallica or letting Ricky Martin's Latin rhythms transport me to the Caribbean. Guaranteed success. These days, I'm able to get mild pain to ease up at home by concentrating on my favourite music. It does, of course, require that I just listen and don't fiddle with anything else. However, live concerts are the best way to enjoy music. The euphoria that comes from a good gig will support me for several days. If my favourite artist happens to be performing nearby, I'll stand on my head in the ticket queue if necessary, without thinking about the pain or anything else.

What you can do

- Do things you like and know how to do. If you have little strength, it's preferable to reinforce an old familiar hobby than to force yourself to try something new.
- At home, concentrate on listening to your favourite music for 20–30 minutes a couple of times a day. It doesn't always have to be something that awakens strong emotions, nor should it be; good basic music is enough. Do this for four weeks and observe the effects.
- There are thousands of free radio channels online (for example, internet-radio.com or tunein.com). You can install an easy-to-use app (such as Spotify or iTunes) on your smartphone, and then you'll always have music with you. If you're having an operation, for instance, take your favourite music along and listen to it on headphones during the procedure.
- Tune in to a dance video on YouTube – perhaps a clip from the film *Sound of Music* or *Jailhouse Rock* by Elvis or *Happy* by Pharrell Williams – close the curtains, and dance yourself into a sweaty, cheerful mood.
- Search online for a recorded concert of your favourite group. Maybe you'll even be inspired to go to a gig.
- If you have even the slightest singing voice, try singing. The health effects of singing haven't been praised without reason. Pluck up your courage and try karaoke at least once in your life. You can take singing lessons online or even join a local choir.
- If you want to try music therapy, trained therapists can be found online (www.bamt.org/). Art therapists can be found here: www.baat.org/
- If pain prevents you from concentrating for more than five minutes at a time, draw on paper or on a tablet with a

drawing program, colour pictures in a colouring book, or listen to an audiobook, which can be borrowed from the library or downloaded from the net, sometimes for free.

- Creative writing courses are offered by many colleges, and groups can also be found online. A notebook on the bedside table or in a tote bag lowers the writing threshold.
- You can set up a book club or even a woodworking club yourself. This is done easily on social media, if you're a social media user otherwise as well. Set up a closed group on Facebook and use it to announce meetings.
- A painting course is a good reason for going abroad, or you can attend one in your own locality. Suitable courses can be found also for beginners.
- Art museums and works by your own favourite artists can be admired online, if the trip to the museum is too long. Operas and band gigs can also be watched on TV and online. A genuine live art experience is, of course, always on a level of its own.

Chapter 18

Consider medication

Treating chronic pain requires time, dedicated effort and a broad mind on the part of both chronic pain patients and the personnel providing treatment. Pharmacological treatment is one aspect of a comprehensive pain toolkit. For some pain patients, drugs are crucial, and for others, they play a minor role, if any. When medications are needed, you and your doctor should carefully consider which pain mechanisms are treated and why.

All long-term treatment, and especially pharmacological treatment, calls for proper information, planning, determination and patience, especially at those times when the new drug does not immediately help or causes unpleasant side-effects. Luckily most side-effects usually pass or ease up with time. Sometimes it takes months to find the right medication. All the hard work and effort put into making a good pain management plan and sticking with it then pays off in providing less pain and suffering, better functioning and, above all, improved quality of life.

Why and when a person living with pain should consider medication

Pain should always be addressed, though not necessarily with medication. Acute pain in particular should not be ignored at the risk of it becoming chronic. Unaddressed pain can disturb and

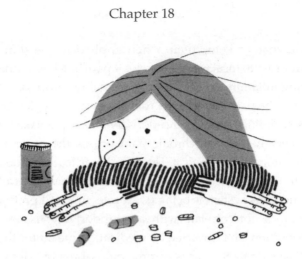

sensitise pain pathways in the nervous system, lowering the pain threshold and making the pain feel more intense in the future. Acute pain often, but not always, calls for pharmacological treatment.

In the case of acute lower back pain – also called lumbago – or pain in the limbs due to strain, the pain can be relieved by taking a non-steroidal anti-inflammatory drug (NSAID) such as ibuprofen (for an adult, 400–800 mg per dose) twice or three times a day for a few days and, in addition, if required, paracetamol (500–1000 mg). A non-steroidal anti-inflammatory drug and paracetamol together for a short period often help better than alone. By contrast, it is not recommended to use two different NSAIDs at the same time since it may increase the risk of adverse effects.

The goal of short-term pharmacological treatment for acute back pain is to reduce the pain to allow normal movement. Staying active and moving are essential for quick recovery. Lying in bed or on the sofa for any length of time may only prolong pain. If your back muscles are very stiff during acute lumbago, you can try a muscle relaxant for the night. However, this isn't essential – relaxants aren't very effective as a whole and they do cause drowsiness. Their long-term use isn't advisable either. Analgesic creams, especially if they contain NSAIDs such as diclofenac or ketoprofen, when applied to the skin may be helpful in acute local musculoskeletal pain, such as tennis elbow, reducing inflammation as part of the healing process.

When the pain persists, the role of pharmacological treatment changes. Ordinary pain medications (NSAIDs, paracetamol) aren't really very helpful for chronic pain unless the cause is clearly inflammatory or mechanical. They work particularly poorly when the pain is centralised, which means that the pain control system of the nervous system is being overprotective and produces pain which does not correlate with any underlying tissue damage. This condition isn't corrected by medication meant for the pain of local tissue damage. Nor is chronic pain of nerve origin, such as impingement on the sciatic nerve or a 'trapped nerve' elsewhere, necessarily eased by NSAIDs.

There are drugs particularly recommended for chronic non-cancer pain. These can influence the mechanisms of chronic pain, not just numb the feeling. You may want to consider those – preferably sooner rather than later – rather than keep taking NSAIDs or even opioids (morphine-like drugs) for years.

What research tells us

In comparison with pharmacological treatment for many other chronic diseases – such as diabetes, asthma, or hypertension – drugs are much less effective for chronic pain. According to recent studies, half of all chronic pain patients don't benefit from pharmacological treatment, and for only about one in three does medication provide enough relief, which is usually around 30-50 per cent reduction in pain intensity. Very rarely 100 per cent pain relief is achieved. For fibromyalgia or chronic low back pain, the effectiveness of pharmacological treatment can be even more modest. In these conditions, better results can be achieved with non-pharmacological alternatives.

One good indication of whether or not medication might be beneficial, or worth continuing, is the 30–30 rule: if on the worst days your pain is 30 per cent less with medication rather than without it, and if there are 30 per cent fewer bad days when taking medication than without it, then medication should be continued. Such an appreciable reduction in pain increases the chronic pain patient's functional capacity, enjoyment and quality of life.

Below I go through some of the most common medications that a GP can prescribe for chronic pain. It isn't possible within the scope of this book to describe in detail all the mechanisms, advantages, disadvantages and combined effects of available medications. Your doctor can tell you more about these. If you know you're allergic to any medication, if you're pregnant, if you have other significant illnesses in addition to your pain symptoms, or if you're already taking other medications, the tips in this book may not necessarily be directly applicable to your situation. It's good to remember that the benefits of any medication are individual. What helps one person isn't necessarily effective for another's pain. In addition, some people can tolerate the side-effects of medications better than others.

The drugs most commonly used to treat chronic pain are:
1.   tricyclic medications (amitriptyline, nortriptyline),
2.   antidepressants that help with pain (serotonin–
      norepinephrine reuptake inhibitors, or 'SNRIs',
      including duloxetine and venlafaxine), and
3.   the anticonvulsants called gabapentinoids (gabapentin,
      pregabalin).

All these drugs relieve pain, for example, by intensifying the functioning of our own pain control systems. One doesn't have to be depressed or epileptic to benefit from them. A GP can prescribe them and expect some benefit.

1. Tricyclics

Tricyclic medications have been in use for decades, so much user experience of them has been built up, and their effects are well known. Originally they were used to treat depression but nowadays they are mostly prescribed for chronic pain. Amitriptyline can improve pain management in many chronic pain states, especially when the pain is associated with a sleep problem. This sort of drug is taken 1–2 hours before bedtime, and it is advisable to start with the lowest possible dose. Then one has to be patient and tolerate feelings of tiredness for a couple of mornings. On about the fourth morning, the medication no longer causes tiredness but may cause a dry mouth. The medication usually improves sleep during the first week, but to improve pain management, the dose usually needs to be increased to 20–25 milligrams over the next couple of weeks. The treatment dose is, however, individual for each person, but for chronic pain is generally a fraction (about 10–30 per cent) of what is prescribed to treat depression.

These medications are usually tolerated quite well, although some people may experience a slowing of bowel function. This side-effect can actually be useful for many who suffer from irritable bowel syndrome (IBS). IBS is a familiar complaint among many chronic pain patients. About 10–20 per cent of the general population suffers from this functional bowel problem which, aside from variations in bowel function, involves bloating and intermittent abdominal pain. People with IBS often have skeletal pain and pain symptoms elsewhere in the body that respond poorly to ordinary analgesics. Examples of these pain symptoms are joint pain, headache and pain in the bladder region.

More has been discovered about IBS-related pain recently. Immune cells, such as monocytes and macrophages, are located in the intestine. The task of these cells is, among other things, to produce morphine-like substances – opioids – needed for pain relief. In a person struggling with an irritable bowel, the immune cell system is disturbed and the production of natural opioids is weakened. In other words, the pain control pathways of the intestinal nerves don't function normally. What's more, the sympathetic nervous system is overactive.

In addition, research indicates that one in three IBS patients also has symptoms of anxiety and/or depression, thus further reinforcing the feeling of pain by altering the process by which the brain handles pain. For many IBS patients, a small dose of tricyclic medicine has a dual effect: the pain threshold is raised and stomach function is calmed. Tricyclic drugs also reduce hyperactivity of the bladder.

2. SNRIs

The SNRI (serotonin–norepinephrine reuptake inhibitors) group of antidepressant medications also prescribed for pain can be helpful for neuropathic and centralised pain. As indicated by their name, these medications can be especially suitable when pain is accompanied by low mood or anxiety. However, pain patients without depression often benefit from them also. The greatest amount of evidence has accumulated for duloxetine, especially in the treatment of neuropathic pain. These SNRI drugs are quite well tolerated, and the dose can be raised quickly – over a week or two – to a suitable level. Sweating, mild headache and nausea, among other side-effects, can occur. Many pain patients benefit from longer courses of treatment, which often last for a few months. During the phase of discontinuing the drug, it is advisable to reduce the dose slowly so that the symptoms associated with stopping (among others, temporary 'jerking' sensations or increased anxiety) are minimised.

3. Gabapentinoids

Gabapentin can relieve the pain of some chronic pain patients, especially when it is associated with a sense of anxiety. One good thing about these drugs is that they have relatively few interactions with other medications. Side-effects, such as dizziness and nausea, can occur, usually when the medication is started. For this reason, the dose should be increased rather slowly. The side-effects usually ease up significantly after a couple of weeks of use.

These drugs were originally developed to treat epilepsy. It makes sense that they also work for chronic pain since chronic pain is known to cause a kind of chaos of electronic signals in the cortex of the brain, as explained at the beginning of the book (Introduction). This is what epilepsy involves as well: uncontrolled electrical activity of the brain and nerve cells. With gabapentin medication, the passing of signals in overactive pain pathways is suppressed and the chaos begins to calm down.

Opioids

Opioids (e.g. codeine, tramadol, buprenorphine, fentanyl, oxycodone, morphine) are used to treat the intense pain symptoms of cancer patients and terminally ill patients, and also to treat pain associated with surgery and/or extensive injuries. For some people living with chronic pain, they can relieve tissue damage-related pain, especially nerve pain symptoms such as sciatica.

The amount of research data on opioids has increased tremendously in recent years, leading to a change in attitudes to their benefits and disadvantages. Their long-term use for chronic, non-cancer-related pain cannot anymore be recommended, at least not as a first-hand treatment and without a comprehensive pain management plan that also includes non-pharmacological treatment modalities, and not without the careful consideration and monitoring of one's own doctor. The introduction of opioids should be left to a doctor who is well informed about pain.

Opioids are a difficult topic, both for chronic pain patients and for doctors. Some patients feel strongly that continuous use of opioids is essential for maintaining their functional capacity and quality of life. Unfortunately, new studies don't support this observation. According to many studies, people who regularly take opioids for their pain seem to cope significantly worse in the longer term than those who treat the same type of pain by other means. People taking opioids experience more fatigue, their daily functional capacity is worse, and depression occurs more often after opioid use has started; this is also the case for sleep problems. The risk of becoming incapacitated for work is greater.

Recent research results on the effects of opioids on sleep are particularly worrying. They break the structure of normal sleep, and can further increase sensitivity to pain and the feeling of fatigue that is associated with it. In the light of current knowledge, opioids may even maintain and worsen pain symptoms, for instance in fibromyalgia, by increasing the sensitivity of the nervous system.

Withdrawal from these medications is difficult. Opioids produce pleasure and increase stress tolerance – more in some, less in others. That's why they are often taken for reasons other than the actual pain symptom. An American pain clinic conducted a study of more than 2000 chronic pain patients, every other one of whom used opioids regularly. The non-depressed pain patients who used opioids took them when the pain became stronger. The depressed pain patients took opioids regardless of what sort of pain they felt. The opioid was taken for symptoms of distress, stress and depression.

Opioids are highly addictive since they have a strong impact on the brain's reward system. Physical and mental dependence develop unfortunately quickly: just five days of opioid use increases the risk of still being on opioids one year later. After 10 days of use, almost one in five will still be taking opioids one year later. In general, the clearer the cause of pain is, the less common it is to develop opioid dependence. Addiction is rarely a problem in treating the pain of cancer, for example. People with concurrent depression and anxiety are at risk of developing dependence partly because both these problems reduce the effectiveness of opioids, in which case the dose can easily become high.

The side-effects associated with opioids are constipation, nausea and changes in hormone balance, such as a decrease in testosterone levels in both women and men. This, in turn, can lead to fatigue, muscle weakness and a lack of sexual desire. The use of opioids lowers cognitive performance and may even increase the risk of dementia, as a recent American study has shown. That particular study looked at 3500 older people who had no symptoms of dementia at the beginning of the research. The risk of developing dementia during the 10-year follow-up period was raised by nearly a third among the older people who used opioids extensively.

Fortunately, research has also yielded convincing evidence that when chronic pain patients slowly stop taking opioids, the pain lessens over time – or at least doesn't get worse. At first there may be withdrawal symptoms, during which time restlessness and the sensation of pain will be heightened, but in the longer term, over the coming weeks and months, life with pain gets easier up, positive emotions return, the quality of sleep improves, fatigue decreases, and there will be scope for other pain management methods.

Migraine

Of all the types of chronic pain, migraine is the one for which medications help best. At the early stages of a migraine attack, an ordinary NSAID at a high enough dose (for instance, 800–1200 mg of ibuprofen taken at a time, or 500–1100 mg of naproxen), or combined with paracetamol, can be helpful for mild migraine. In addition, the anti-nausea medication metoclopramide, which accelerates the absorption of the analgesic, can be taken.

Migraine pain is one of the strongest neurological pains a person can experience. Targeted drugs called triptans have been developed to treat more intense migraine. These affect the potential cause of migraine by binding to serotonin receptors in the brain to diminish the swelling of blood vessels. Fortunately, triptans work well for most patients. The pain is relieved within 30 minutes to two hours after being taken. There are no great differences between the various triptan preparations available.

For chronic migraine or regular attacks, topiramate, propranolol or amitriptyline can be used as preventive medication.

Codeine or other opioids are not recommended for treating a migraine attack. They only block the pain signals for a few hours, and don't affect the mechanism giving rise to migraine. The headache returns, often stronger than before. Opioids are used for migraine only if the patient doesn't tolerate other medications, or if the triptans together with an NSAID or paracetamol don't help.

Melatonin

Studies done on the neurotransmitter and hormone melatonin have shown that it may also have a place in pain management. Melatonin is the naturally occurring 'night hormone' in the body. It is secreted by the pineal gland in the brain. In fibromyalgia, melatonin alone or in combination with amitriptyline has brought pain relief. According to one study on endometriosis pain – which is a relatively common cause for pain in the pelvic region among women – daily pain decreased with high dose of melatonin (10 mg) for eight weeks by 40 per cent, and the need for analgesics decreased by 80 per cent. It would seem that melatonin raises the pain threshold of healthy people as well. It supports sleep and reduces anxiety, both of which usually benefit people living with chronic pain. Melatonin has been used for instance before surgery, to relieve the associated tension. Its effectiveness has been found to be of the order of the sedative tranquilisers, benzodiazepines. Melatonin is a relatively safe preparation; its side-effects are at the level of a placebo and it doesn't appreciably cause addiction.

Naltrexone

Low-dose naltrexone would appear in some cases to work for fibromyalgia and CFS. Studies conducted, among others, at the renowned Stanford University have found that this drug works well for some people, while others don't benefit from it at all. Naltrexone has an interesting mechanism of action: it blocks opioid receptors for a short time. The daily dose is usually 3–5 mg. The same medication is used, in doses about 10 times greater, to treat alcohol and opioid addiction.

Many medications meant for pain relief only act through one mechanism. Chronic pain often originates from local tissue damage or the peripheral nervous system, as well as from the central nervous system. That's why combining several different medications can be beneficial. The back pain patient who has suffered from sciatica for a long time may benefit from the following combination (if pharmacological treatment is needed): paracetamol and/or an NSAID for pain flares plus a longer course of an antidepressant also prescribed for pain, such as duloxetine, to calm the pain pathways and intensify the functioning of his/ her own pain control mechanisms. Occasionally, a modest dose of opioids for 1-3 days is needed for chronic pain flare-ups and/ or neuropathic pain symptoms.

My own experience

My experience of working with patients

Both patients and doctors often have unrealistic expectations about the effectiveness of medications. I myself never recommend only pharmacological treatment for pain, especially if the pain is chronic and has begun to control the patient's life. Non-pharmacological modalities are definitely needed as well.

Many people with chronic pain have a lowered tolerance and increased sensitivity to the side-effects of medications. They also often have other diseases and take many medications for them; possible interactions should always be taken into account. Adjusting medication involves balancing between adequate effectiveness and tolerating side-effects.

Many of the pain patients I treat – ordinary working people – have a negative attitude to medications. People shy away from the unpleasant side-effects of medications for pain: drowsiness, nausea, heartburn and constipation. They are also afraid that these medications may cause addiction. They may be ashamed of pain medication, in the same way as they are ashamed of their pain. Many people living with chronic pain report feeling that the doctor or pharmacist considers them 'junkies' if they have to take opioids. Patients tell me that being labelled as a 'drug addict' feels like an additional punishment in life.

I'm concerned about the pharmacological treatment of chronic pain patients. One of my worries is that too many try to treat their chronic pain with NSAIDs. These medications don't alleviate the pain well, but they are still taken despite the risk of a gastric ulcer and heart disease. I believe many think there is no other option. Also, antidepressants that are useful for chronic pain are not prescribed early enough, or for long enough periods. I often hear my patients say that they don't want medication because they don't think they're depressed. This is one of the misunderstandings that I hope reading this book will change. You need not be depressed to benefit from an antidepressant.

Another of my worries pertains to opioids. The tremendous increase in the number of opioid prescriptions in the Western world (including Britain) doesn't indicate an improvement in pain management, rather quite the opposite. My concern is associated with the fact that to control unpleasant pain and relieve stress, people try to numb their pain system with heavy painkillers. Then, when effective pain management is truly needed – for instance, in connection with an accident – the medication for that acute pain may not be effective enough. Also, knowledge of the disadvantages of opioids, such as poorer sleep quality, hasn't spread widely enough. I'm also concerned about the combined use of opioids with other medications, such as benzodiazepines, or with alcohol. A person who takes opioids should definitely avoid alcohol and sedatives.

The most serious opioid-related adverse event is reduced respiratory function. Every year, hundreds of ordinary people

– those who are not considered to be drug addicts – die at night of respiratory failure caused by prescription opioids. This isn't talked about enough, in my opinion.

Every chronic pain patient deserves the best possible evidence-based, personally-tailored care. Pharmacological treatment should be discussed honestly. In particular, the benefits and disadvantages of regular use of opioids should be reviewed and all of the methods for improving pain management considered so that the use of opioids can be minimised – or even discontinued altogether. This book includes almost 20 of these methods. Such an approach is in the best interests of everyone living with chronic pain. Cancer-related pain is a separate matter that I won't address here.

Managing my own pain

I manage my own pain mainly by non-pharmacological methods, and I cope quite well. If necessary I take ibuprofen, and sometimes paracetamol as well. A migraine attack requires a triptan.

Some chronic pain medications have been beneficial for me for other pains. The difficult worsening phase of sciatic pain has sometimes required codeine. I try to avoid using it since the feeling it brings with it is an unpleasant listless tipsiness. If I've had to take codeine in the evening, in the morning I've noticed I'm in a state of 'brain fog', with memory gaps and slow thinking. Thus for my part, opioid medication mostly sits in my medicine cabinet and I'm satisfied that I don't much need it.

In the past, at times, I've taken a two- to three-week course of melatonin, in doses of 3–6 mg taken in the evening. As a result, my headaches have diminished and I've slept well – but I have been a lively dreamer.

At this point, I'd like to point out that I've written this book without any financial commitments to the pharmaceutical industry or any other part of the pain management business!

What you can do

- Many people have great expectations of medication and may be bitterly disappointed if it doesn't help right away or doesn't alleviate the pain completely. Talk about your medication with your doctor and, above all, be patient. Sometimes it takes months or even years before suitable pharmacological treatment is found.
- Nearly every medication pack has a long list of side-effects because the law requires the inclusion of even very rare symptoms that some person may have experienced. Don't be frightened when reading the list. Most of the possible side-effects probably won't affect you but do, of course, be aware of any that do arise and consult your doctor.
- Many people's opinions and experiences of medications can be found online. Many of these are the outbursts of disappointed people needing to vent their frustration. Keep in mind that people who are doing well are less likely to write about their positive experiences online.

Appendices

Appendix 1

Things you can influence yourself – and how they affect pain

Optimism

Friends, other social support

Mood

Positivity

An open mind

Sleep

Enthusiasm

The courage to do things despite pain

Shifting attention away from pain

Identifying fears associated with pain

Accurate information

Positive expectations of life despite pain

Appendix 1

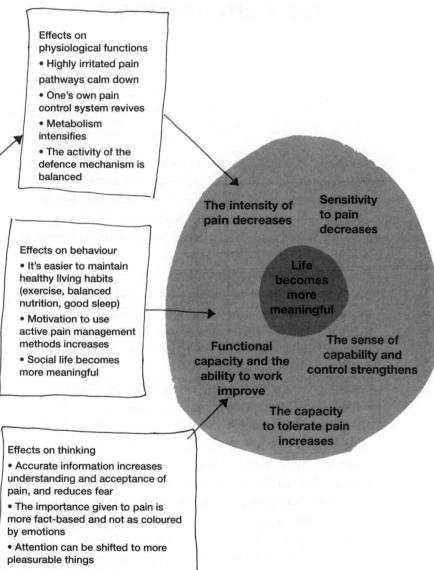

Effects on physiological functions
• Highly irritated pain pathways calm down
• One's own pain control system revives
• Metabolism intensifies
• The activity of the defence mechanism is balanced

Effects on behaviour
• It's easier to maintain healthy living habits (exercise, balanced nutrition, good sleep)
• Motivation to use active pain management methods increases
• Social life becomes more meaningful

Effects on thinking
• Accurate information increases understanding and acceptance of pain, and reduces fear
• The importance given to pain is more fact-based and not as coloured by emotions
• Attention can be shifted to more pleasurable things
• Thinking becomes more flexible

The intensity of pain decreases

Sensitivity to pain decreases

Life becomes more meaningful

The sense of capability and control strengthens

Functional capacity and the ability to work improve

The capacity to tolerate pain increases

Appendix 2

Work arrangements

The following are suggestions for work arrangements that can help a person suffering from pain cope at work better. If you are the pain sufferer, share this with your boss/line manager and be aware, depending on your national legislation, it is likely your employer is obliged by law to approach your work situation in this way.

- Flexible use of time: try tailor-made working hours and/or flexitime; avoid overnight shifts and long shifts; allow for breaks, for instance long weekends, by using holiday time
- Regular breaks: allow for time-out/rest/catnaps that are long enough to relax and preferably not in the person's own office/desk/work site
- Consider the possibility of working remotely and of switching off from work during free time
- Give some control: if it's possible, allow the pain sufferer to manage their own work content, order and use of time
- Think flexibly: consider what the pain sufferer is capable of and adjust what they do to maximise what they can bring to the job; avoid physically heavy tasks or provide adequate assistance when they have to be done; try working in pairs; vary tasks through job rotation
- Tech help: provide lifting devices, ergonomic tools and other technical auxiliary devices
- IT support: provide a larger computer screen, speech

recognition software

- Postural support: consider whether it would help to provide a roller mouse, a better office chair, an electrically adjustable desk or a platform, a saddle chair, an exercise ball instead of an office chair, suitable lighting, computer glasses, other ergonomic auxiliary devices
- Personal work equipment: the pain sufferer may benefit from good work shoes, warm, flexible clothing, protective gloves, trolleys and bags, protective goggles
- Environmental conditions: all workers will benefit from fresh indoor air, a steady work temperature and reduction of draughts
- Peaceful working area: ensure the pain sufferer has peace to concentrate, the possibility of listening to music if this won't interfere with the job, noise protection devices (noise-cancelling headphones, etc.)
- Mobility issues: move the person to a work site closer to the social facilities, coffee room and toilet; provide a parking place near the entrance
- Avoid or reduce work-related travel
- Sufficient induction: provide sufficient support if the pain sufferer takes on new, different work or returns to their former work after a long sick leave; induction may be needed for the adoption of new computer software or changes in work practices
- Transparency: the pain sufferer needs a clear job description, the support of their immediate superior, and peer support in the work community
- Time out for health support: give the pain sufferer permission to take the time they need to care for their health and maintain their ability to work; ensure they have a peaceful area for talking with the nurse or doctor over the phone
- Good supervision: ensure the pain sufferer has regular meetings with their line manager and can have open and

encouraging discussions so trust can be built
- Understanding colleagues: provide information and guidance for the work community so they can support a colleague living with chronic pain and not feel that person is getting preferential treatment
- Foster a positive spirit in the work community: this can be done through fair play, respect, greeting others, distribution of information, helping others, joint coffee breaks, Christmas parties, exercise breaks, mindfulness breaks, yoga classes.

Note for pain sufferers working in the UK

In the UK, The Equality Act 2010 obliges the employer to make 'reasonable adjustments' so that employees disabled by chronic pain, as well as other problems, are not discriminated against or put at a disadvantage. The definition of 'reasonable adjustments' is not specified but the measures listed above are very much the sorts of accomodation the employer has to consider to help the employee continue to work.

Sources of advice and information about this and the rights of the disabled employee include:
- ACAS: for employers – www.employeradvice.org/ACAS-Code; for employees – www.acas.org.uk/disability
- the Equality Commission – https://equalityhumanrights.com
- the CAB – www.citizensadvice.org.uk/law-and-courts/discrimination/protected-characteristics/showing-you-re-disabled-under-the -equality-act/

Appendix 3

What the pain sufferer needs from you

This guidance is for partners, friends and co-workers of sufferers from chronic pain and for anyone reporting to them in the workplace.

For a partner

For someone living with chronic pain, pain is almost always present in one form or another. On good days the pain isn't necessarily forgotten, and on bad days it overrides almost everything else. When your family's holiday plans are cancelled because of your partner's pain and fatigue, or when you as the healthier adult have to do more housework than your partner who suffers from pain, it's natural that feelings of irritation or anger rise to the surface at times. Or that they do so when at bad moments your partner is absorbed in him/herself, isn't communicative, avoids interaction and jumps when touched. A hug may feel unpleasant, even painful, and the mere thought of sex may be too much for your partner.

You may feel frustrated or guilty that you aren't able to do more to ease your partner's discomfort. You may hide your feelings of helplessness and your own exhaustion because you think that you have to be strong and the member of the family who can cope.

It's important for you to accept that you can't solve your partner's situation, as there is no one solution. Nor should you take on too much responsibility for your partner's doings, or do too much on his/her behalf, because it's likely that you'll become exhausted yourself. Then there would be two weary people in your relationship.

Instead, use your strength to learn to provide the kind of support that actually benefits your partner who is living with pain. S/he appreciates your help even if s/he doesn't always know how, or have the strength, to express it. Just listening and being present – especially in bad times – is of great importance.

Chronic pain is a very personal issue. It can cause a huge sense of loneliness. It's good to remember that our in-built defence mechanisms may sometimes work against our wellbeing: they may lead us to curl up around our pain and isolate ourselves from others. It is very common for a chronic pain patient to say that s/he is a burden to his/her partner and family. The pain sufferer may decide that s/he no longer wants to burden loved ones with his/her pain and discomfort. In general, this only leads to deepening of the discomfort and deterioration of the situation. Learn to recognise your partner's unspoken communication and to notice when his/her pain is getting worse. Take a moment then to help him/her rest, or give him/her a hug, if s/he wishes; stroke him/her and be close. Encourage him/her to talk about how s/he is feeling, and about his/her pain.

At the same time, learn to tell your partner how you are feeling, and also talk about your frustration and/or feelings of helplessness. Do it constructively and calmly. Your partner who is living with pain will surely want to know your thoughts and feelings instead of just guessing them. This will encourage him/her to talk about his/her own feelings as well. It will help to create an open and close relationship between the two of you, which in itself is a huge source of strength for coping with pain.

It's important that your spirits stay positive even if your

partner is caught up in a heavy or depressed emotional state and focuses these feelings on you or blames you. This is a common and human, partly unconscious, defence reaction among people who are tired; don't take it personally. When your partner has rested and is a little less fatigued, tell him/her how important it is, in spite of everything, to see the positive in the situation and in your life together. Tell him/her the good things that you appreciate. Think together about which of the helpful, enjoyable, pleasure-producing things described in this book your partner could do so that s/he would be able to manage his/her pain better, while at the same time remaining active. You can do them together, simultaneously inspiring and encouraging each other. On better days there's more strength to be active, and activity in turn brings more of the better days.

Accompany your partner to the doctor's at least once so that you get more information about pain and your partner's situation. There are peer support groups for the immediate family of chronic pain patients – groups which provide information and support. Remember also to look after your own health and wellbeing, and try to find some time for yourself, to do things you enjoy.

For a friend

Everyone living with pain wishes s/he could live pain free, or even just have a life where the next day would in some way be predictable. However, one feature of chronic pain is that the symptoms may worsen unexpectedly, without any particular reason. At such times, your friend who's living with chronic pain may cancel get-togethers and other arrangements. Even if this has happened, do ask your friend to join you again – and again. S/he probably appreciates it very much even if s/he doesn't know how to express it. It's important for a person living with chronic pain to experience being a desirable companion even if s/he isn't always able to participate. Loneliness is worse than feeling guilty for not being able to meet friends as often as one would like. Agree to stay in touch also by phone or online. Don't be offended if your friend living with chronic pain lacks the strength to speak on the phone or communicate online when you contact him/her.

Many friends and family members experience helplessness in the face of pain. A person who isn't in pain can't understand how chronic pain feels and how it affects life. Even though it isn't possible to understand fully the other person's situation, you can still provide support. Ask your friend what kind of support and help s/he would need for good days and bad days. Try to maintain your own positive and encouraging attitude. You shouldn't look for and suggest reasons for your friend's pain, since it's rare to find a single cause for chronic pain. If a solution for eliminating pain were available, your friend surely would have found it already. It's therefore worth considering the timing of, and the need for, suggestions and advice. Acceptance, listening and presence work best.

When you spend time together, learn to note signs that the pain is worsening: restlessness, irritability, inability to concentrate, messages conveyed by facial expressions, gritting the teeth. If you see these signs, ask your friend how s/he feels, if the pain is getting worse, and what you could do to relieve this. A short break in your current activities may then be a good idea, so that your friend can rest, relax and, if necessary, take medication.

It can be surprisingly simple to find good alternatives for spending time together. Your friend may not be able to play badminton anymore, but s/he might be delighted by an invitation to play table tennis. Or a card game. Or instead of the traditional all-day bargain hunting, you could spend a couple of hours shopping followed by pampering at a spa. A week's holiday in the sun could be replaced by a weekend trip to a mindfulness retreat. The most important thing is to spend time together. Humour and laughing together are good ways to empower us and forget pain. Stand-up comedy works really well. It can be watched together online if your friend isn't up to going to a live gig. Or send your friend a link to a sweet cat video. Kittens bumbling about – it works every time.

For a co-worker

Chronic pain usually doesn't show on the surface, no matter how miserable a person may be feeling. Your co-worker who suffers from chronic pain doesn't necessarily talk about his/her condition or situation at the workplace, and at bad times s/he may avoid social encounters. Not speaking to others isn't necessarily because the chronic pain sufferer doesn't want to talk about his/her issues, or doesn't trust you. It's just that s/he can't always find the words to describe his/her symptoms and condition. S/he may need to withdraw from coffee-time conversations about travel experiences or what happened at a Christmas party. As important as these social breaks are to the atmosphere at work, on bad days a person living with chronic pain can't identify with gaiety. Just getting out of bed that morning may have been a big deal for him/her.

The person living with chronic pain generally appreciates being asked about his/her situation in private, and at a peaceful time convenient to him/her. There's no need to lament or be sad about anything, or to offer solutions; a matter-of-fact, calm attitude and acceptance are enough. Ask whether it would be good to tell other members of the workforce some essential facts about the nature of chronic pain, and more generally how pain affects everyday performance (without necessarily mentioning anything personal). Understanding and acceptance increase with the right information. Respect your co-worker's wishes also if s/he doesn't want anything about his/her situation known in the workplace.

For your co-worker, going to work is probably a much healthier alternative than struggling with pain symptoms alone at home. Think together about how the work could be adapted, and tasks shared so that the person with chronic pain would be able to manage at work. On particularly bad days, the support of the work community is invaluable. On better days, the person with chronic pain may have the strength and enthusiasm to do even too much, which in turn can lead to a worsening of pain on the next few days.

Every one of us has times in life when our health acts up, and the ability to work can be reduced temporarily. At such times, we need the support of our co-workers. That's why it's good to learn to be flexible and to show empathy towards co-workers with a reduced ability to work, so that we ourselves would get the same kind of support when we need it.

For a boss or line manager

As a manager, you will surely have to face one of the biggest challenges of anyone in a supervisory position: how to deal with a worker plagued by health problems, such as chronic pain and fatigue, and how to support his/her ability and work. It's understandable if you find it so difficult that it's easier not to bring up the whole issue at all, preferring to advise the worker to go on sick leave. Some managers may be in the habit of forbidding the worker to come back to work until the pain symptoms have disappeared completely and ability to work has returned to 100 per cent.

However, health and the ability to work aren't an either–or situation of 0 per cent or 100 per cent where the person can be defined as either completely healthy or really ill, either fully capable or totally disabled. Health and the ability to work fall on a continuum that has an endless number of permutations with the person moving between them. A person's own experience of his/her health or ability to work can be situated at a point on this continuum that is completely different from the doctor's or manager's opinion of it. Nevertheless, our society is largely built round this on–off thinking. This is one of the most important reasons why so many chronic pain sufferers drift into disability. How the worker him/herself experiences his/her situation is a very strong predictor of what will happen to him/her in the future. It pays to listen to him/her.

In Chapter 10, Keep working, I go into more detail about how chronic pain affects work, and how work affects chronic pain. According to the present view, continuing at work despite chronic pain, or similar, maintains and promotes health. Waiting passively at home rarely improves chronic pain symptoms, while exclusion from work and working life may even worsen the condition. The most important thing is to find the right kind of work and suitable hours that the worker can handle, and that would provide the best support for his/her pain management and health.

There are days and periods when, understandably, work isn't the first thing on the mind of a person struggling with investigations, diagnosis, medication trials, insomnia, fatigue and lack of strength. At such times, the person is occupied with merely surviving from one day to the next. On the other hand, if the person has to give up working altogether for a long time, recovering the ability to work and returning to it can be an impossible battle.

The duties and responsibilities of a manager include supporting the chronic pain patient's ability to work whenever work arrangements and other work-related support measures allow. (In the UK, we have seen employers are obliged under The Equality Act to make 'reasonable adjustments'; what these might be needs to be discussed with the pain sufferer.) As a smart manager, you should learn how to recognise and take account of the worsening symptoms of the worker reporting to you, as well as fluctuations in functioning and the ability to work. Encourage him/her to talk about his/her situation. Together you can discuss what temporary modifications and flexibilities would enable him/her to cope at work. You can make use of the suggestions on work arrangements presented in Appendix 2.

Chronic pain eats away at the sufferer's strength and self-esteem. As the manager, you have the opportunity to both maintain and support your worker's positive work identity and self-esteem in a significant way. Give him/her feedback that s/he is doing good work and is a valued worker despite his/her chronic health problem, if this is the case.

Communicate to the worker that the workplace you lead is one of openness and trust. It is advisable to train and instruct the workforce to support the health and ability to work of the worker with chronic pain. A negative or sceptical attitude among workers usually reflects lack of information, or worry. You can ask an occupational health professional to tell your workforce about pain and work-related issues. Perhaps a peer support person who would help the worker with chronic pain can be found from within the workforce itself. There are good experiences of such activities, for example, in Norway, where research results on the topic have been published. Peer support at the place of work would even seem to reduce overall sick leave.

Psychological support is important, but that alone isn't enough if it isn't seen as producing concrete results. Together with the worker who has chronic pain, draw up a plan of work arrangements that could be tried, and when and how you'll follow the plan's implementation. Make use of the expertise of occupational health personnel, especially an occupational physiotherapist. If support measures fall short, try something else. The worker is the best expert in his/her own work, so it's important to hear his/her thoughts. Remember also to look after your own coping and, if necessary, to seek support and information for yourself from occupational health professionals. The work of a manager calls for training and coaching, and what has been learned should be updated repeatedly. It pays to make the effort, because your training is directly reflected in the wellbeing of both you and your workers.

References

Preface; Introduction: A new understanding of pain; Chapter 1: Get the right information; Appendices

Apkarian AV, Hashmi JA, Baliki MN. Pain and the brain: specificity and plasticity of the brain in clinical chronic pain. *Pain* 2011; 152: S49-64. doi: 10.1016/j.pain.2010.11.010.

Arendt-Nielsen L, Morlion B, Perrot S, Dahan A, Dickenson A, Kress HG, Wells C, Bouhassira D, Mohr Drewes A. Assessment and manifestation of central sensitisation across different chronic pain conditions. *European Journal of Pain* 2018; 22: 216-241. doi: 10.1002/ejp.1140.

Berryman C, Stanton TR, Bowering JK, Tabor A, McFarlane A, Moseley LG. Evidence for working memory deficits in chronic pain: a systematic review and meta-analysis. *Pain* 2013; 154: 1181-96. doi: 10.1016/j.pain.2013.03.002.

Breivik H, Collett B, Ventafridda V, Cohen R, Gallacher D. Survey of chronic pain in Europe: prevalence, impact on daily life, and treatment. *European Journal of Pain* 2006; 10: 287-333. (also referred in Chapters 4: Don't underestimate the power of touch, and 10: Keep working)

Bresler D. Raising pain tolerance using guided imagery. *Practical Pain Management* 2010; 10: 6.

Butler D, Moseley LG. *Explain Pain* 2nd edition. Noigroup Publications 2013.

Carriere JS, Sturgeon JA, Yakobov E, Kao MC, Mackey SC, Darnall BD. The impact of perceived injustice on pain-related outcomes: a combined model examining the mediating roles of pain acceptance and anger in a chronic pain sample. *Clinical Journal of Pain* 2018; 34: 739-747. doi: 10.1097/ajp.0000000000000602. (Also referred in Chapter 6: Talk about your feelings)

Darlow B, Forster BB, O'Sullivan K, O'Sullivan P. It is time to stop causing harm with inappropriate imaging for low back pain. *British Journal of Sports Medicine* 2017; 51: 414-415. doi: 10.1136/bjsports-2016-096741

deCharms RC, Maeda F, Glover GH, Ludlow D, Pauly JM, Soneji D, Gabrieli JD, Mackey SC. Control over brain activation and pain learned by using real-time functional MRI. *Proceedings of the National Academy of Sciences of the United States of America* 2005; 102: 18626-18631. (Also referred in Chapters 5: Do what you enjoy, and 9: Experience the power of mindfulness)

Edwards RR, Cahalan C, Mensing G, Smith M, Haythornthwaite JA. Pain, catastrophizing, and depression in the rheumatic diseases. *Nature Reviews Rheumatology* 2011; 7: 216-24. doi: 10.1038/nrrheum.2011.2.

Farioli A, Mattioli S, Quaglieri A, Curti S, Violante FS, Coggon D. Musculoskeletal pain in Europe: role of personal, occupational and social risk factors. *Scandinavian Journal of Work, Environment & Health* 2014; 40: 36-46. doi: 10.5271/sjweh.3381.

Fingleton C, Smart K, Moloney N, Fullen BM, Doody C. Pain sensitization in people with knee osteoarthritis: a systematic review and meta-analysis. *Osteoarthritis and Cartilage* 2015; 23: 1043-1056. doi: 10.1016/j.joca.2015.02.163.

Galambos A, Szabó E, Nagy Z, Édes AE, Kocsel N, Juhász G, Kökönyei G. A systematic review of structural and functional MRI studies on pain catastrophizing. *Journal of Pain Research* 2019; 12: 1155-1178. doi: 10.2147/JPR.S192246.

Grice-Jackson T, Critchley HD, Banissy MJ, Ward J. Consciously feeling the pain of others reflects atypical functional connectivity between the pain matrix and frontal-parietal regions. *Frontiers in Human Neuroscience* 2017; 11: 507. doi: 10.3389/fnhum.2017.00507.

Hartvigsen J, Hancock MJ, Kongsted A, Louw Q, Ferreira ML, Genevay S, Hoy D, Karppinen J, Pransky G, Sieper J, Smeets RJ,

References

Underwood M; Lancet Low Back Pain Series Working Group. What low back pain is and why we need to pay attention. *Lancet* 2018; 391: 2356-2367. doi: 10.1016/S0140-6736(18)30480-X.

Hurwitz EL, Randhawa K, Yu H, Côté P, Haldeman S. The Global Spine Care Initiative: a summary of the global burden of low back and neck pain studies. *European Spine Journal* 2018; 27: S6: 796-801. doi: 10.1007/s00586-017-5432-9.

Jackson T, Wang Y, Wang Y, Fan H. Self-efficacy and chronic pain outcomes: a meta-analytic review. *Journal of Pain* 2014; 15: 800-14. doi: 10.1016/j.jpain.2014.05.002.

Job Accommodation Network – https://askjan.org/ (Accessed 16 June 2019)

Karasawa Y, Yamada K, Iseki M, Yamaguchi M, Murakami Y, Tamagawa T, Kadowaki F, Hamaoka S, Ishii T, Kawai A, Shinohara H, Yamaguchi K, Inada E. Association between change in self-efficacy and reduction in disability among patients with chronic pain. *PLoS One* 2019; 14: e0215404. doi: 10.1371/journal.pone.0215404.

Koyama T, McHaffie JG, Laurienti PJ, Coghill RC. The subjective experience of pain: where expectations become reality. *Proceedings of the National Academy of Sciences USA* 2005; 102: 12950-2955.

Kregel J, Meeus M, Malfliet A, Dolphens M, Danneels L, Nijs J, Cagnie B. Structural and functional brain abnormalities in chronic low back pain: a systematic review. *Seminars in Arthritis and Rheumatism* 2015; 45: 229-37. doi: 10.1016/j.semarthrit.2015.05.002.

Kress HG, Aldington D, Alon E, Coaccioli S, Collett B, Coluzzi F, Huygen F, Jaksch W, Kalso E, Kocot-Kępska M, Mangas AC, Ferri CM, Mavrocordatos P, Morlion B, Müller-Schwefe G, Nicolaou A, Hernández CP, Sichère P. A holistic approach to chronic pain management that involves all stakeholders: change is needed. *Current Medical Research and Opinion* 2015; 31: 1743-54. doi: 10.1185/03007995.2015.1072088.

Kurita GP, Sjøgren P, Juel K, Højsted J, Ekholm O. The burden of chronic pain: a cross-sectional survey focussing on diseases, immigration, and opioid use. *Pain* 2012; 153: 2332-8. doi: 10.1016/j.pain.2012.07.023.

Lee H, Hübscher M, Moseley GL, Kamper SJ, Traeger AC, Mansell G, McAuley JH. How does pain lead to disability? A systematic

review and meta-analysis of mediation studies in people with back and neck pain. *Pain* 2015; 156: 988-97.
doi: 10.1097/j.pain.0000000000000146.

Li G, Abbade LPF, Nwosu I, Jin Y, Leenus A, Maaz M, Wang M, Bhatt M, Zielinski L, Sanger N, Bantoto B, Luo C, Shams I1, Shahid H, Chang Y, Sun G, Mbuagbaw L, Samaan Z, Levine MAH , Adachi JD, Thabane L. A systematic review of comparisons between protocols or registrations and full reports in primary biomedical research. *BMC Medical Research Methodology* 2018; 18: 9.
doi: 10.1186/s12874-017-0465-7.

McCluskey S, de Vries H, Reneman M, Brooks J, Brouwer S. 'I think positivity breeds positivity': a qualitative exploration of the role of family members in supporting those with chronic musculoskeletal pain to stay at work. *BMC Family Practice* 2015; 16: 85.
doi: 10.1186/s12875-015-0302-1.

Miranda H, Gold JE, Gore R, Punnett L. Recall of prior musculoskeletal pain. *Scandinavian Journal of Work, Environment and Health* 2006; 32: 294-299.

Ng SK, Urquhart DM, Fitzgerald PB, Cicuttini FM, Hussain SM, Fitzgibbon BM. The relationship between structural and functional brain changes and altered emotion and cognition in chronic low back pain brain changes: a systematic review of MRI and fMRI studies. *Clinical Journal of Pain* 2018; 34: 237-261.
doi: 10.1097/AJP.0000000000000534.

Nijs J, Malfliet A, Ickmans K, Baert I, Meeus M. Treatment of central sensitization in patients with 'unexplained' chronic pain: an update. *Expert Opinion on Pharmacotherapy* 2014; 15: 1671-83.
doi: 10.1517/14656566.2014.925446. (also referred in Chapter 18, Consider medication)

Ojala T. The essence of the experience of chronic pain – A phenomenological study. Doctoral dissertation. University of Jyväskylä, Finland 2015.

Olaya-Contreras P. Bio-psychosocial analyses of acute and chronic pain, especially in the spine – the effect of distress on pain intensity and disability. Doctoral dissertation. University of Gothenburg, Sweden 2011.

Osborn J, Derbyshire SW. Pain sensation evoked by observing injury in others. *Pain* 2010; 148: 268-274. doi: 10.1016/j.pain.2009.11.007.

Raspe H, Hueppe A, Neuhauser H. Back pain, a communicable disease? *International Journal of Epidemiology* 2008; 37: 69-74.

Robertson O, Robinson SJ, Stephens R. Swearing as a response to pain: A cross-cultural comparison of British and Japanese participants. *Scandinavian Journal of Pain* 2017; 17: 267-272. doi: 10.1016/j.sjpain.2017.07.014.

Steffens D, Hancock MJ, Maher CG, Williams C, Jensen TS, Latimer J. Does magnetic resonance imaging predict future low back pain? A systematic review. *European Journal of Pain* 2014; 18: 755–65. doi: 10.1002/j.1532-2149.2013.00427.x.

Stephens R, Atkins J, Kingston A. Swearing as a response to pain. *Neuroreport* 2009; 20: 1056-60. doi: 10.1097/WNR.0b013e32832e64b1.

Story GW, Vlaev I, Seymour B, Winston JS, Darzi A, Dolan RJ. Dread and the disvalue of future pain. *PLoS Computational Biology* 2013; 9: e1003335. doi: 10.1371/journal.pcbi.1003335.

Thompson EL, Broadbent J, Bertino MD, Staiger PK. Do pain-related beliefs influence adherence to multidisciplinary rehabilitation? A systematic review. *Clinical Journal of Pain* 2016; 32: 164-178. doi: 10.1097/AJP.0000000000000235.

Tonosu J, Oka H, Higashikawa A, Okazaki H, Tanaka S, Matsudaira K. The associations between magnetic resonance imaging findings and low back pain: A 10-year longitudinal analysis. *PLoS One* 2017; 12: e0188057. doi: 10.1371/journal.pone.0188057.

Chapter 2: Value your sleep

Afolalu EF, Ramlee F, Tang NKY. Effects of sleep changes on pain-related health outcomes in the general population: A systematic review of longitudinal studies with exploratory meta-analysis. *Sleep Medicine Reviews* 2018; 39: 82-97. doi: 10.1016/j.smrv.2017.08.001.

Aili K, Nyman T, Svartengren M, Hillert L. Sleep as a predictive factor for the onset and resolution of multi-site pain: a 5-year prospective study. *European Journal of Pain* 2015; 19: 341-349. doi: 10.1002/ejp.552.

Aili K, Andersson M, Bremander A, Haglund E, Larsson I, Bergman

S. Sleep problems and fatigue as predictors for the onset of chronic widespread pain over a 5- and 18-year perspective. *BMC Musculoskeletal Disorders* 2018; 19: 390. doi: 10.1186/s12891-018-2310-5.

Alsaadi SM, McAuley JH, Hush JM, Lo S, Lin CW, Williams CM, Maher CG. Poor sleep quality is strongly associated with subsequent pain intensity in patients with acute low back pain. *Arthritis & Rheumatology* 2014; 66: 1388-1394. doi: 10.1002/art.38329.

Burgess HJ, Burns JW, Buvanendran A, Gupta R, Chont M, Kennedy M, Bruehl S. Associations between sleep disturbance and chronic pain intensity and function: a test of direct and indirect pathways. *Clinical Journal of Pain* 2019; 35(7): 569-576. doi: 10.1097/AJP.0000000000000711.

Campbell CM, Buenaver LF, Finan P, Bounds SC, Redding M, McCauley L, Robinson M, Edwards RR, Smith MT. Sleep, pain catastrophizing, and central sensitization in knee osteoarthritis patients with and without insomnia. *Arthritis Care & Research* 2015; 67: 1387-1396. doi: 10.1002/acr.22609.

Canadian Agency for Drugs and Technologies in Health. *Mattresses for chronic back or neck pain: a review of the clinical effectiveness and guidelines.* 2014. Ottawa (ON): Canadian Agency for Drugs and Technologies in Health; 2014 May. https://www.ncbi.nlm.nih.gov/books/NBK263379/ (accessed 16 June 2019)

Charokopos A, Card ME, Gunderson C, Steffens C, Bastian LA. The association of obstructive sleep apnea and pain outcomes in adults: a systematic review. *Pain Medicine* 2018; 19: S69-S75. doi: 10.1093/pm/pny140.

Correa D, Farney RJ, Chung F, Prasad A, Lam D, Wong J. Chronic opioid use and central sleep apnea: A review of the prevalence, mechanisms, and perioperative considerations. *Anesthesia and Analgesia* 2015; 120: 1273-1285. doi: 10.1213/ANE.0000000000000672.

Curtis AF, Miller MB, Boissoneault J, Robinson M, Staud R, Berry RB, McCrae CS. Discrepancies in sleep diary and actigraphy assessments in adults with fibromyalgia: Associations with opioid dose and age. *Journal of Sleep Research* 2018: e12746. doi: 10.1111/jsr.12746.

Curtis AF, Miller MB, Rathinakumar H, Robinson M, Staud R, Berry

References

RB, McCrae CD. Opioid use and sleep architecture in fibromyalgia. *Sleep* 2019; 42: S1: A339–A340.

Diaz-Piedra C, Di Stasi LL, Baldwin CM, Buela-Casal G, Catena A. Sleep disturbances of adult women suffering from fibromyalgia: A systematic review of observational studies. *Sleep Medicine Reviews* 2015; 21: 86–99. doi: 10.1016/j.smrv.2014.09.001.

Dimsdale JE, Norman D, DeJardin D, Wallace MS. The effect of opioids on sleep architecture. *Journal of Clinical Sleep Medicine* 2007; 3: 33.

Filiatrault ML, Chauny JM, Daoust R, Roy MP, Denis R, Lavigne G. Medium increased risk for central sleep apnea but not obstructive sleep apnea in long-term opioid users: a systematic review and meta-analysis. *Journal of Clinical Sleep Medicine* 2016; 12: 617-625. doi: 10.5664/jcsm.5704.

Finan PH, Goodin BR, Smith MT. The association of sleep and pain: An update and a path forward. *Journal of Pain* 2013; 14: 1539-1552. doi: 10.1016/j.jpain.2013.08.007.

Huang CT, Chiang RP, Chen CL, Tsai YJ. Sleep deprivation aggravates median nerve injury-induced neuropathic pain and enhances microglial activation by suppressing melatonin secretion. *Sleep* 2014; 37: 1513-1523. doi: 10.5665/sleep.4002.

Koffel E, McCurry S, Smith MT, Vitiello MV. Improving pain and sleep in middle-aged and older adults: the promise of behavioral sleep interventions. *Pain* 2019; 160: 529-534. doi: 10.1097/j.pain.0000000000001423.

Krause AJ, Prather AA, Wager TD, Lindquist MA, Walker MP. The pain of sleep loss: a brain characterization in humans. *Journal of Neuroscience* 2019; 39: 2291-2300. doi: 10.1523/jneurosci.2408-18.2018.

Linder J, Jansen GB, Ekholm KS, Ekholm J. Relationship between sleep disturbance, pain, depression and functioning in long-term sick-listed patients experiencing difficulty in resuming work. *Journal of Rehabilitation Medicine* 2014; 46: 798-805. doi: 10.2340/16501977-1833.

McBeth J, Lacey RJ, Wilkie R. Predictors of new-onset widespread pain in older adults: results from a population-based prospective cohort study in the UK. *Arthritis & Rheumatology* 2014; 66: 757-767. doi: 10.1002/art.38284.

Merikanto I, Lahti T, Seitsalo S, Kronholm E, Laatikainen T, Peltonen

M, Vartiainen E, Partonen T. Behavioral trait of morningness-eveningness in association with articular and spinal diseases in a population. *PLoS One* 2014; 9: e114635. doi: 10.1371/journal.pone.0114635.

Miranda H, Viikari-Juntura E, Punnett L, Riihimäki H. Occupational loading, health behavior and sleep disturbance as predictors of low back pain. *Scandinavian Journal of Work, Environment and Health* 2008; 34: 411-419.

Mork PJ, Nilsen TI. Sleep problems and risk of fibromyalgia: longitudinal data on an adult female population in Norway. *Arthritis & Rheumatology* 2012; 64: 281-284. doi: 10.1002/art.33346.

Roth T, Bhadra-Brown P, Pitman VW, Resnick EM. Pregabalin improves fibromyalgia-related sleep disturbance. *Clinical Journal of Pain* 2016; 32: 308-312. doi: 10.1097/ajp.0000000000000262.

Simpson NS, Scott-Sutherland J, Gautam S, Sethna N, Haack M. Chronic exposure to insufficient sleep alters processes of pain habituation and sensitization. *Pain* 2018; 159: 33-40. doi: 10.1097/j.pain.0000000000001053.

Sivertsen B, Lallukka T, Petrie KJ, Steingrímsdóttir ÓA, Stubhaug A, Nielsen CS. Sleep and pain sensitivity in adults. *Pain* 2015; 156: 1433-1439. doi: 10.1097/j.pain.0000000000000131.

Tang NK, Lereya ST, Boulton H, Miller MA, Wolke D1, Cappuccio FP. Nonpharmacological treatments of insomnia for long-term painful conditions: a systematic review and meta-analysis of patient-reported outcomes in randomized controlled trials. *Sleep* 2015; 38: 1751-64. doi: 10.5665/sleep.5158.

Wei Y, Blanken TF, Van Someren EJW. Insomnia really hurts: effect of a bad night's sleep on pain increases with insomnia severity. *Frontiers in Psychiatry* 2018; 9: 377. doi: 10.3389/fpsyt.2018.00377.

Chapter 3: Discover the importance of positive thinking

Catalino LI, Algoe SB, Fredrickson BL. Prioritizing positivity: An effective approach to pursuing happiness? *Emotion* 2014; 14: 1155-1161. doi: 10.1037/a0038029.

Cogan R, Cogan D, Waltz W, McCue M. Effects of laughter and

relaxation on discomfort thresholds. *Journal of Behavioral Medicine* 1987; 10: 139–144.

Dunbar RI, Baron R, Frangou A, Pearce E, van Leeuwen EJ, Stow J, Partridge G, MacDonald I, Barra V, van Vugt M. Social laughter is correlated with an elevated pain threshold. *Proceedings of the Royal Society B: Biological Sciences* 2012; 279: 1161-1167. doi: 10.1098/rspb.2011.1373.

Esteve R, López-Martínez AE, Peters ML, Serrano-Ibáñez ER, Ruiz-Párraga GT, Ramírez-Maestre C. Optimism, positive and negative affect, and goal adjustment strategies: their relationship to activity patterns in patients with chronic musculoskeletal pain. *Pain Research and Management* 2018; 6291719. doi: 10.1155/2018/6291719.

Finan PH, Garland EL. The role of positive affect in pain and its treatment. *Clinical Journal of Pain* 2015; 31: 177-187.

Finlay F, Baverstock A, Lenton S. Therapeutic clowning in paediatric practice. *Clinical Child Psychology and Psychiatry* 2014; 19: 596-605. doi: 10.1177/1359104513492746.

Goodin BR, Glover TL, Sotolongo A, King CD, Sibille KT, Herbert MS, Cruz-Almeida Y, Sanden SH, Staud R, Redden DT, Bradley LA, Fillingim RB. The association of greater dispositional optimism with less endogenous pain facilitation is indirectly transmitted through lower levels of pain catastrophizing. *Journal of Pain* 2013; 14: 126-135. doi: 10.1016/j.jpain.2012.10.007.

Graham-Engeland JE, Zawadzki MJ, Slavish DC, Smyth JM. Depressive symptoms and momentary mood predict momentary pain among rheumatoid arthritis patients. *Annals of Behavioral Medicine* 2016; 50: 12-23. doi: 10.1007/s12160-015-9723-2.

Hanssen MM, Peters ML, Vlaeyen JW, Meevissen YM, Vancleef LM. Optimism lowers pain: evidence of the causal status and underlying mechanisms. *Pain* 2012; 154: 53-58. doi: 10.1016/j.pain.2012.08.006.

Hanssen MM. Optimism, the natural placebo. Cognitive, behavioural and motivational mechanisms of resilience towards pain. Doctoral dissertation. Maastricht: University of Maastricht, the Netherlands, 2014.

Hanssen MM, Peters ML, Boselie JJ, Meulders A. Can positive affect attenuate (persistent) pain? State of the art and clinical

implications. *Current Rheumatology Reports* 2017; 19: 80.
doi: 10.1007/s11926-017-0703-3.

Kahneman D, Tversky A. Choices, values, and frames. *American Psychologist* 1984; 39:3 41-50. doi: 10.1037/0003-066X.39.4.341

Kamping S, Bomba IC, Kanske P, Diesch E, Flor H. Deficient modulation of pain by a positive emotional context in fibromyalgia patients. *Pain* 2013; 154: 1846-1855. doi: 10.1016/j.pain.2013.06.003.

Keeris D. Chronic pain and positive emotions: A systematic review. Doctoral dissertation. University of Twente, the Netherlands, 2015.

Nummenmaa L, Tuominen L. Opioid system and human emotions. *British Journal of Pharmacology* 2018; 175: 2737-2749. doi: 10.1111/bph.13812.

Malfliet A, Coppieters I, Van Wilgen P, Kregel J, De Pauw R, Dolphens M, Ickmans K. Brain changes associated with cognitive and emotional factors in chronic pain: A systematic review. *European Journal of Pain* 2017; 21: 769-786. doi: 10.1002/ejp.1003.

Manninen S, Tuominen L, Dunbar RI, Karjalainen T, Hirvonen J, Arponen E, Hari R, Jääskeläinen IP, Sams M, Nummenmaa L. Social laughter triggers endogenous opioid release in humans. *Journal of Neuroscience* 2017; 37: 6125-6131. doi: 10.1523/jneurosci.0688-16.2017.

Pérez-Aranda A, Hofmann J, Feliu-Soler A, Ramírez-Maestre C, Andrés-Rodríguez L, Ruch W, Luciano JV. Laughing away the pain: A narrative review of humour, sense of humour and pain. *European Journal of Pain* 2019; 23: 220-233. doi: 10.1002/ejp.1309.

Robinson H, Norton S, Jarrett P, Broadbent E. The effects of psychological interventions on wound healing: A systematic review of randomized trials. *British Journal of Health Psychology* 2017; 22: 805-835. doi: 10.1111/bjhp.12257.

Romundstad S, Svebak S, Holen A, Holmen J. A 15-year follow-up study of sense of humor and causes of mortality: the Nord-Trøndelag Health Study. *Psychosomatic Medicine* 2016; 78: 345-353. doi: 10.1097/psy.0000000000000275.

Rotton J, Shats M. Effects of state humor, expectancies, and choice on postsurgical mood and self-medication: a field experiment. *Journal of Applied Social Psychology* 1996; 26: 1775–1794.

Van Cappellen P, Rice EL, Catalino LI, Fredrickson BL. Positive affective processes underlie positive health behaviour change. *Psychology &*

Health 2018; 33: 77-97. doi: 10.1080/08870446.2017.1320798.

Vilaythong AP, Arnau RC, Rosen DH, Mascaro N. Humor and hope: Can humor increase hope? *International Journal of Humor Research* 2006; 16: 79-89. doi.org/10.1515/humr.2003.006

Chapter 4: Don't underestimate the power of touch

Ahn SJ, Kyeong S, Suh SH, Kim JJ, Chung TS, Seok JH. What is the impact of child abuse on gray matter abnormalities in individuals with major depressive disorder: a case control study. *BMC Psychiatry* 2016; 16: 397. doi: 10.1186/s12888-016-1116-y

Assefi N, Bogart A, Goldberg J, Buchwald D. Reiki for the treatment of fibromyalgia: a randomized controlled trial. *Journal of Alternative and Complementary Medicine* 2008; 14: 1115-1122. doi: 10.1089/acm.2008.0068.

Billot M, Daycard M, Wood C, Tchalla A. Reiki therapy for pain, anxiety and quality of life. *BMJ Supportive & Palliative Care* 2019. Published online 4 April 2019. doi: 10.1136/bmjspcare-2019-001775.

Caruso S, Mauro D, Scalia G, Palermo CI, Rapisarda AMC, Cianci A. Oxytocin plasma levels in orgasmic and anorgasmic women. *Gynecological Endocrinology* 2018; 34: 69-72. doi: 10.1080/09513590.2017.1336219.

Descalzi G, Ikegami D, Ushijima T, Nestler EJ, Zachariou V, Narita M. Epigenetic mechanisms of chronic pain. *Trends in Neuroscience* 2015; 38: 237-246. doi: 10.1016/j.tins.2015.02.001.

Edmiston EE, Wang F, Mazure CM, Guiney J, Sinha R, Mayes LC, Blumberg HP. Corticostriatal-limbic gray matter morphology in adolescents with self-reported exposure to childhood maltreatment. *Archives of Pediatrics and Adolescent Medicine* 2011; 165: 1069-1077. doi: 10.1001/archpediatrics.2011.565.

Furlan AD, Giraldo M, Baskwill A, Irvin E, Imamura M. Massage for low-back pain. *Cochrane Database of Systematic Reviews* 2015; CD001929. doi: 10.1002/14651858.CD001929.pub3.

Gentile D, Boselli D, O'Neill G, Yaguda S, Bailey-Dorton C, Eaton TA. Cancer pain relief after healing touch and massage. *Journal of*

Alternative and Complementary Medicine 2018; 24: 968-973.
doi: 10.1089/acm.2018.0192.

Giannitrapani K, Holliday J, Miake-Lye I, Hempel S, Taylor SL.
Synthesizing the strength of the evidence of complementary and
integrative health therapies for pain. *Pain Medicine* 2019; pnz068.
doi: 10.1093/pm/pnz068.

Hambach A, Evers S, Summ O, Husstedt IW, Frese A. The impact of
sexual activity on idiopathic headaches: an observational study.
Cephalalgia 2013; 33: 384-389. doi: 10.1177/0333102413476374.

Hudson BF, Ogden J, Whiteley MS. Randomized controlled trial to
compare the effect of simple distraction interventions on pain and
anxiety experienced during conscious surgery. *European Journal of
Pain* 2015, 19: 1447-1455. doi: 10.1002/ejp.675.

Jong TR, Menon R, Bludau A, Grund T, Biermeier V, Klampfl SM,
Jurek B, Bosch OJ, Hellhammer J, Neumann ID. Salivary oxytocin
concentrations in response to running, sexual self-stimulation,
breastfeeding and the TSST: The Regensburg Oxytocin Challenge
(ROC) study. *Psychoneuroendocrinology* 2015; 62: 381-388.
doi: 10.1016/j.psyneuen.2015.08.027.

Li YH, Wang FY, Feng CQ, Yang XF, Sun YH. Massage therapy
for fibromyalgia: a systematic review and meta-analysis of
randomized controlled trials. *PLoS One* 2014; 20: e89304.
doi: 10.1371/journal.pone.0089304.

Mancini F, Nash T, Iannetti GD, Haggard P. Pain relief by touch: A
quantitative approach. *Pain* 2014; 155: 635–42.
doi: 10.1016/j.pain.2013.12.024.

Miake-Lye IM, Mak S, Lee J, Luger T, Taylor SL, Shanman R, Beroes-
Severin JM, Shekelle PG. Massage for pain: an evidence map.
Journal of Alternative and Complementary Medicine 2019; 25: 475-502.
doi: 10.1089/acm.2018.0282.

Shin ES, Seo KH, Lee SH, Jang JE, Jung YM, Kim MJ, Yeon JY. Massage
with or without aromatherapy for symptom relief in people with
cancer. *Cochrane Database of Systematic Reviews* 2016; CD009873.
doi: 10.1002/14651858.CD009873.pub3.

Skelly AC, Chou R, Dettori JR, Turner JA, Friedly JL, Rundell SD, Fu
R, Brodt ED, Wasson N, Winter C, Ferguson AJR. Noninvasive
nonpharmacological treatment for chronic pain: a systematic
review. *Comparative Effectiveness Review No. 209*. (Prepared by the

Pacific Northwest Evidence-based Practice Center under Contract No. 290-2015-00009-I.) AHRQ Publication No 18-EHC013-EF. Rockville, MD: Agency for Healthcare Research and Quality; June 2018. doi: https://doi.org/10.23970/ahrqepccer209

So PS, Jiang Y, Qin Y. Touch therapies for pain relief in adults. *Cochrane Database of Systematic Reviews* 2008; CD006535. doi: 10.1002/14651858.CD006535.pub2.

Whipple B, Komisaruk BR. Elevation of pain threshold by vaginal stimulation in women. *Pain* 1985; 21: 357-367.

Wise NJ, Frangos E, Komisaruk BR. Brain activity unique to orgasm in women: An fMRI analysis. *Journal of Sexual Medicine* 2017; 14: 1380-1391. doi: 10.1016/j.jsxm.2017.08.014.

Youssef NA, Lockwood L, Su S, Hao G, Rutten BPF. The effects of trauma, with or without PTSD, on the transgenerational DNA methylation alterations in human offsprings. *Brain Sciences* 2018; 8. doi: 10.3390/brainsci8050083.

Yuan SL, Matsutani LA, Marques AP. Effectiveness of different styles of massage therapy in fibromyalgia: a systematic review and meta-analysis. *Manual Therapy* 2015; 20: 257-264. doi: 10.1016/j.math.2014.09.003.

Chapter 5: Do what you enjoy

Spoil yourself

Antonelli M, Donelli D. Effects of balneotherapy and spa therapy on levels of cortisol as a stress biomarker: a systematic review. *International Journal of Biometeorology* 2018; 62: 913-924. doi: 10.1007/s00484-018-1504-8.

Bazzichi L, Da Valle Y, Rossi A, Giacomelli C, Sernissi F, Giannaccini G, Betti L, Ciregia F, Giusti L, Scarpellini P, Dell'Osso L, Marazziti D, Bombardieri S, Lucacchini A. A multidisciplinary approach to study the effects of balneotherapy and mud-bath therapy treatments on fibromyalgia. *Clinical and Experimental Rheumatology* 2013; 31: 6: S111-20.

Chary-Valckenaere I, Loeuille D, Jay N, Kohler F, Tamisier JN, Roques CF, Boulange M, Gay G. Spa therapy together with supervised self-mobilisation improves pain, function and quality of life in patients with chronic shoulder pain: a single-blind randomised controlled trial. *International Journal of Biometeorology* 2018; 62: 1003-1014. doi: 10.1007/s00484-018-1502-x.

Fioravanti A, Cantarini L, Guidelli GM, Galeazzi M. Mechanisms of action of spa therapies in rheumatic diseases: what scientific evidence is there? *Rheumatology International* 2011; 31: 1-8. doi: 10.1007/s00296-010-1628-6.

Fraioli A, Mennuni G, Fontana M, Nocchi S, Ceccarelli F, Perricone C, Serio A. Efficacy of spa therapy, mud-pack therapy, balneotherapy, and mud-bath therapy in the management of knee osteoarthritis. A systematic review. *BioMed Research International* 2018; 1042576. doi: 10.1155/2018/1042576.

Honigman L, Bar-Bachar O, Yarnitsky D, Sprecher E, Granovsky Y. Nonpainful wide-area compression inhibits experimental pain. *Pain* 2016; 157: 2000-2011. doi: 10.1097/j.pain.0000000000000604.

Karagülle M, Karagülle MZ. Effectiveness of balneotherapy and spa therapy for the treatment of chronic low back pain: a review on latest evidence. *Clinical Rheumatology* 2015; 34: 207-214. doi: 10.1007/s10067-014-2845-2.

Karagülle M, Kardeş S, Karagülle O, Dişçi R, Avcı A, Durak İ, Karagülle MZ. Effect of spa therapy with saline balneotherapy on oxidant/antioxidant status in patients with rheumatoid arthritis: a single-blind randomized controlled trial. *International Journal of Biometeorology* 2017; 61: 169-180. doi: 10.1007/s00484-016-1201-4.

Karagülle M, Kardeş S, Karagülle MZ. Long-term efficacy of spa therapy in patients with rheumatoid arthritis. *Rheumatology International* 2018; 38: 353-362. doi: 10.1007/s00296-017-3926-8.

Mooventhan A, Nivethitha L. Scientific evidence-based effects of hydrotherapy on various systems of the body. *North American Journal of Medicine & Science* 2014; 6: 199–209. doi: 10.4103/1947-2714.132935

Naumann J, Sadaghiani C. Therapeutic benefit of balneotherapy and hydrotherapy in the management of fibromyalgia syndrome: a qualitative systematic review and meta-analysis of randomized controlled trials. *Arthritis Research & Therapy* 2014; 16: R141. doi: 10.1186/ar4603.

Perrot S, Russell IJ. More ubiquitous effects from non-pharmacologic than from pharmacologic treatments for fibromyalgia syndrome:

References

A meta-analysis examining six core symptoms. *European Journal of Pain* 2014; 18: 1067–1080. doi: 10.1002/ejp.564.

Tenti S, Cheleschi S, Galeazzi M, Fioravanti A. Spa therapy: can be a valid option for treating knee osteoarthritis? *International Journal of Biometeorology* 2015; 59: 1133-1143. doi: 10.1007/s00484-014-0913-6.

Verhagen AP, Bierma-Zeinstra SM, Boers M, Cardoso JR, Lambeck J, de Bie R, de Vet HC. Balneotherapy (or spa therapy) for rheumatoid arthritis. *Cochrane Database of Systematic Reviews* 2015; CD000518. doi: 10.1002/14651858.CD000518.pub2.

Visualise your 'soul's landscape'

Bowering KJ, O'Connell NE, Tabor A, Catley MJ, Leake HB, Moseley GL, Stanton TR. The effects of graded motor imagery and its components on chronic pain: a systematic review and meta-analysis. *Journal of Pain* 2013; 14: 3-13. doi: 10.1016/j.jpain.2012.09.007.

Fardo F, Allen M, Jegindø EM, Angrilli A, Roepstorff A. Neurocognitive evidence for mental imagery-driven hypoalgesic and hyperalgesic pain regulation. *Neuroimage* 2015; 120: 350-361. doi: 10.1016/j.neuroimage.2015.07.008.

Hansen MM, Jones R, Tocchini K. Shinrin-Yoku (Forest Bathing) and Nature Therapy: A State-of-the-Art Review. *International Journal of Environmental Research and Public Health* 2017; 14: 851. doi: 10.3390/ijerph14080851.

Jensen KB, Berna C, Loggia ML, Wasan AD, Edwards RR, Gollub RL. The use of functional neuroimaging to evaluate psychological and other non-pharmacological treatments for clinical pain. *Neuroscience Letters* 2012; 520: 156-164. doi: 10.1016/j.neulet.2012.03.010.

Mygind L, Kjeldsted E, Hartmeyer RD, Mygind E, Bølling M, Bentsen P. Immersive nature-experiences as health promotion interventions for healthy, vulnerable, and sick populations? A systematic review and appraisal of controlled studies. *Frontiers in Psychology* 2019; 10: 943. doi: 10.3389/fpsyg.2019.00943.

Nørgaard MW, Werner A, Abrahamsen R, Larsen B, Darmer MR, Pedersen PU. Visualization and attentive behavior for pain reduction during radiofrequency ablation of atrial fibrillation.

Pacing and Clinical Electrophysiology 2013; 36: 203-213.
doi: 10.1111/pace.12032.

Zech N, Hansen E, Bernardy K, Häuser W. Efficacy, acceptability and safety of guided imagery/hypnosis in fibromyalgia – A systematic review and meta-analysis of randomized controlled trials. *European Journal of Pain* 2017; 21: 217-227. doi: 10.1002/ejp.933.

Maintain social relationships

Anastas TM, Meints SM, Gleckman AD, Hirsh AT. Social influences on peer judgments about chronic pain and disability. *Journal of Pain* 2018 Dec 21. doi: 10.1016/j.jpain.2018.12.006.

Cacioppo S, Balogh S, Cacioppo JT. Implicit attention to negative social, in contrast to nonsocial, words in the Stroop task differs between individuals high and low in loneliness: evidence from event-related brain microstates. *Cortex* 2015; 70: 213-233. doi: 10.1016/j.cortex.2015.05.032.

Chan TH. Facebook and its effects on users' empathic social skills and life satisfaction: a double-edged sword effect. *Cyberpsychology, Behavior, and Social Networking* 2014; 17: 276-280. doi: 10.1089/cyber.2013.0466.

Cole SW, Hawkley LC, Arevalo JM, Sung CY, Rose RM, Cacioppo JT. Social regulation of gene expression in human leukocytes. *Genome Biology* 2007; 8: R189. doi: 10.1186/gb-2007-8-9-r189

Ferrari R. Effect of a pain diary use on recovery from acute low back (lumbar) sprain. *Rheumatology International* 2014; 35: 55-59. doi: 10.1007/s00296-014-3082-3.

Hadert A, Rodham K. The invisible reality of arthritis: a qualitative analysis of an online message board. *Musculoskeletal Care* 2008; 6: 181-196. doi: 10.1002/msc.131.

Holt-Lunstad J, Smith TB, Layton JB. Social relationships and mortality risk: a meta-analytic review. *PLoS Medicine* 2010; 7: e1000316. doi: 10.1371/journal.pmed.1000316.

Kostova Z, Caiata-Zufferey M, Schulz PJ. Can social support work virtually? Evaluation of rheumatoid arthritis patients' experiences with an interactive online tool. *Pain Research & Management* 2015; 20: 199-209.

Lapidot-Lefler N, Barak A. Effects of anonymity, invisibility, and lack of eye-contact on toxic online disinhibition. *Computers in Human Behavior* 2012; 28: 434-443. doi: 10.1016/j.chb.2011.10.014

Merolli M, Gray K, Martin-Sanchez F. Health outcomes and related effects of using social media in chronic disease management: A literature review and analysis of affordances. *Journal of Biomedical Informatics* 2013; 46: 957-969. doi: 10.1016/j.jbi.2013.04.010.

Nowland R, Necka EA, Cacioppo JT. Loneliness and social internet use: pathways to reconnection in a digital world? *Perspectives on Psychological Science* 2018; 13: 70-87. doi: 10.1177/1745691617713052.

Shiovitz-Ezra S, Parag O. Does loneliness 'get under the skin'? Associations of loneliness with subsequent change in inflammatory and metabolic markers. *Aging & Mental Health* 2018: 1-9. doi: 10.1080/13607863.2018.1488942.

Smith TO, Dainty JR, Williamson E, Martin KR. Association between musculoskeletal pain with social isolation and loneliness: analysis of the English Longitudinal Study of Ageing. *British Journal of Pain* 2019; 13:82-90. doi: 10.1177/2049463718802868.

Yin J, Lassale C, Steptoe A, Cadar D. Exploring the bidirectional associations between loneliness and cognitive functioning over 10 years: the English longitudinal study of ageing. *International Journal of Epidemiology* 2019 May 5. doi: 10.1093/ije/dyz085.

Ziebland S, Wyke S. Health and illness in a connected world: how might sharing experiences on the internet affect people's health? *Milbank Quarterly* 2012; 90: 219- 249. doi: 10.1111/j.1468-0009.2012.00662.x

Play

Gupta A, Scott K, Dukewich M. Innovative technology using virtual reality in the treatment of pain: does it reduce pain via distraction, or is there more to it? *Pain Medicine* 2018; 19: 151-159. doi: 10.1093/pm/pnx109.

Jameson E, Trevena J, Swain N. Electronic gaming as pain distraction. *Pain Research and Management* 2011; 16: 27-32.

Keefe FJ, Huling DA, Coggins MJ, Keefe DF, Zachary Rosenthal M, Herr NR, Hoffman HG. Virtual reality for persistent pain: A new direction for behavioral pain management. *Pain* 2012; 153: 2163–2166. doi: 10.1016/j.pain.2012.05.030.

Wiederhold BK, Gao K, Sulea C, Wiederhold MD. Virtual reality as a distraction technique in chronic pain patients. *Cyberpsychology, Behavior, and Social Networking* 2014;17:346–352. doi: 10.1089/cyber.2014.0207.

Wittkopf PG, Lloyd DM, Coe O, Yacoobali S, Billington J. The effect of interactive virtual reality on pain perception: a systematic review of clinical studies. *Disability and Rehabilitation* 2019 May 8: 1-12. doi: 10.1080/09638288.2019.1610803.

Relax

Dunford E. Relaxation and mindfulness in pain: A review. *Reviews in Pain* 2010; 4: 18-22.

Jeffrey S, McClelland T, Carus C, Graham C. Relaxation and chronic pain: A critical review. *International Journal of Therapy and Rehabilitation* 2016; 23: 6. doi: 10.12968/ijtr.2016.23.6.289

Kim HS, Kim EJ. Effects of relaxation therapy on anxiety disorders: a systematic review and meta-analysis. *Archives of Psychiatric Nursing* 2018; 32: 278-284. doi: 10.1016/j.apnu.2017.11.015.

Klainin-Yobas P, Oo WN, Suzanne Yew PY, Lau Y. Effects of relaxation interventions on depression and anxiety among older adults: a systematic review. *Aging & Mental Health* 2015; 19: 1043-1055. doi: 10.1080/13607863.2014.997191.

Kropp P, Meyer B, Meyer W, Dresler T. An update on behavioral treatments in migraine – current knowledge and future options. *Expert Review of Neurotherapeutics* 2017; 17: 1059-1068. doi: 10.1080/14737175.2017.1377611.

Kwekkeboom KL, Gretarsdottir E. Systematic review of relaxation interventions for pain. *Journal of Nursing Scholarship* 2006; 38: 269-277.

Meyer B, Keller A, Wöhlbier HG, Overath CH, Müller B, Kropp P. Progressive muscle relaxation reduces migraine frequency and normalizes amplitudes of contingent negative variation (CNV). *Journal of Headache and Pain* 2016; 17: 37. doi: 10.1186/s10194-016-0630-0.

Rota E, Evangelista A, Ceccarelli M, Ferrero L, Milani C, Ugolini A, Mongini F. Efficacy of a workplace relaxation exercise program on muscle tenderness in a working community with headache and neck pain: a longitudinal, controlled study. *European Journal of Physical and Rehabilitation Medicine* 2016; 52: 457-465.

Theadom A, Cropley M, Smith HE, Feigin VL, McPherson K. Mind and body therapy for fibromyalgia. *Cochrane Database of Systematic Reviews* 2015; CD001980. doi: 10.1002/14651858.CD001980.pub3.

Zhang Y, Montoya L, Ebrahim S, Busse JW, Couban R, McCabe RE, Bieling P, Carrasco-Labra A, Guyatt GH. Hypnosis/relaxation therapy for temporomandibular disorders: a systematic review and meta-analysis of randomized controlled trials. *Journal of Oral & Facial Pain and Headache* 2015; 29: 115-125. doi: 10.11607/ofph.1330.

Chapter 6: Talk about your feelings

Aaron RV, Fisher EA, de la Vega R, Lumley MA, Palermo TM. Alexithymia in individuals with chronic pain and its relation to pain intensity, physical interference, depression, and anxiety: a systematic review and meta-analysis. *Pain* 2019; 160: 994-1006. doi: 10.1097/j.pain.0000000000001487.

Berna C, Leknes S, Holmes EA, Edwards RR, Goodwin GM, Tracey I. Induction of depressed mood disrupts emotion regulation neurocircuitry and enhances pain unpleasantness. *Biological Psychiatry* 2010; 67: 11: 1083-1090. doi: 10.1016/j.biopsych.2010.01.014.

Burns JW, Gerhart JI, Bruehl S, Post KM, Smith DA, Porter LS, Schuster E, Buvanendran A, Fras AM, Keefe FJ. Anger arousal and behavioral anger regulation in everyday life among patients with chronic low back pain: relationships to patient pain and function. *Health Psychology* 2016; 35: 29-40. doi: 10.1037/hea0000221.

Ferdousi M, Finn DP. Stress-induced modulation of pain: role of the endogenous opioid system. *Progress in Brain Research* 2018; 239: 121-177. doi: 10.1016/bs.pbr.2018.07.002.

Galvez-Sánchez CM, Reyes Del Paso GA, Duschek S. Cognitive impairments in fibromyalgia syndrome: associations with positive and negative affect, alexithymia, pain catastrophizing and self-esteem. *Frontiers in Psychology* 2018; 9: 377. doi: 10.3389/fpsyg.2018.00377.

Hughes LS, Clark J, Colclough JA, Dale E, McMillan D. Acceptance and Commitment Therapy (ACT) for chronic pain: A systematic review and meta-analyses. *Clinical Journal of Pain.* 2017; 33: 552-568. doi: 10.1097/ajp.0000000000000425.

IsHak WW, Wen RY, Naghdechi L, Vanle B, Dang J, Knosp M, Dascal J, Marcia L, Gohar Y, Eskander L, Yadegar J, Hanna S, Sadek A, Aguilar-Hernandez L, Danovitch I, Louy C. Pain and depression: a systematic review. *Harvard Review of Psychiatry* 2018; 26: 352-363. doi: 10.1097/hrp.0000000000000198.

Kamping S, Bomba IC, Kanske P, Diesch E, Flor H. Deficient modulation of pain by a positive emotional context in fibromyalgia patients. *Pain* 2013; 154: 1846-1855. doi: 10.1016/j.pain.2013.06.003.

Koechlin H, Coakley R, Schechter N, Werner C, Kossowsky J. The role of emotion regulation in chronic pain: A systematic literature review. *Journal of Psychosomatic Research* 2018; 107: 38-45. doi: 10.1016/j.jpsychores.2018.02.002.

Kowal J, Wilson KG, McWilliams LA, Péloquin K, Duong D. Self-perceived burden in chronic pain: relevance, prevalence, and predictors. *Pain* 2012; 153: 1735– 1741. doi: 10.1016/j.pain.2012.05.009.

Lumley MA, Schubiner H. Emotional awareness and expression therapy for chronic pain: rationale, principles and techniques, evidence, and critical review. *Current Rheumatology Reports* 2019; 21: 30. doi: 10.1007/s11926-019-0829-6.

Martinez-Calderon J, Flores-Cortes M, Morales-Asencio JM, Luque-Suarez A. Pain-related fear, pain intensity and function in individuals with chronic musculoskeletal pain: a systematic review and meta-analysis. *Journal of Pain* 2019 May 4. doi: 10.1016/j.jpain.2019.04.009

Pinheiro MB, Ferreira ML, Refshauge K, Ordoñana JR, Machado GC, Prado LR, Maher CG, Ferreira PH. Symptoms of depression and risk of new episodes of low back pain. A systematic review and meta-analysis. *Arthritis Care and Research* (Hoboken) 2015; 67: 1591-1603. doi: 10.1002/acr.22619.

Poole H, White S, Blake C, Murphy P, Bramwell R. Depression in chronic pain patients: prevalence and measurement. *Pain Practice* 2009; 9: 173-180. doi: 10.1111/j.1533-2500.2009.00274.x.

Rayner L, Hotopf M, Petkova H, Matcham F, Simpson A, McCracken

LM. Depression in patients with chronic pain attending a specialised pain treatment centre: prevalence and impact on health care costs. *Pain* 2016; 157: 1472–1479. doi: 10.1097/j.pain.0000000000000542

Richmond H, Hall AM, Copsey B, Hansen Z, Williamson E, Hoxey-Thomas N, Cooper Z, Lamb SE. The effectiveness of cognitive behavioural treatment for non-specific low back pain: a systematic review and meta-analysis. *PLoS One* 2015; 10: e0134192. doi: 10.1371/journal.pone.0134192

Sullivan MJ, Scott W, Trost Z. Perceived injustice: a risk factor for problematic pain outcomes. *Clinical Journal of Pain* 2012; 28: 484-488. doi: 10.1097/AJP.0b013e3182527d13.

Viana MC, Lim CCW, Garcia Pereira F, Aguilar-Gaxiola S, Alonso J, Bruffaerts R, de Jonge P, Caldas-de-Almeida JM, O'Neill S, Stein DJ, Al-Hamzawi A, Benjet C, Cardoso G, Florescu S, de Girolamo G, Haro JM, Hu C, Kovess-Masfety V, Levinson D, Piazza M, Posada-Villa J, Rabczenko D, Kessler RC, Scott KM. Previous mental disorders and subsequent onset of chronic back or neck pain: findings from 19 countries. *Journal of Pain* 2018; 19: 99-110. doi: 10.1016/j.jpain.2017.08.011.

Zale EL, Lange KL, Fields SA, Ditre JW. The relation between pain-related fear and disability: a meta-analysis. *Journal of Pain* 2013; 14: 1019–1030. doi: 10.1016/j.jpain.2013.05.005.

Chapter 7: Eat wisely

Agarwal KA, Tripathi CD, Agarwal BB, Saluja S. Efficacy of turmeric (curcumin) in pain and postoperative fatigue after laparoscopic cholecystectomy: a double-blind, randomized placebo-controlled study. *Surgical Endoscopy* 2011; 25: 3805-3810. doi: 10.1007/s00464-011-1793-z.

Bagis S, Karabiber M, As I, Tamer L, Erdogan C, Atalay A. Is magnesium citrate treatment effective on pain, clinical parameters and functional status in patients with fibromyalgia? *Rheumatology International* 2013; 33: 167-172. doi: 10.1007/s00296-011-2334-8.

Beasley M, Freidin MB, Basu N, Williams FMK, Macfarlane GJ. What is the effect of alcohol consumption on the risk of chronic widespread pain? A Mendelian randomisation study using UK Biobank. *Pain* 2019; 160: 501-507. doi: 10.1097/j.pain.0000000000001426.

Branton WG, Ellestad KK, Maingat F, Wheatley BM, Rud E, Warren RL, Holt RA, Surette MG, Power C. Brain microbial populations in HIV/AIDS: α-proteobacteria predominate independent of host immune status. *PLoS One* 2013; 8: e54673. doi: 10.1371/journal.pone.0054673.

Cameron M, Chrubasik S. Topical herbal therapies for treating osteoarthritis. *Cochrane Database of Systematic Reviews* 2013: CD010538. doi: 10.1002/14651858.cd010538.

Castaner O, Goday A, Park YM, Lee SH, Magkos F, Shiow STE, Schröder H. The gut microbiome profile in obesity: a systematic review. *International Journal of Endocrinology* 2018; 2018: 4095789. doi: 10.1155/2018/4095789.

Chen S, Roffey DM, Dion CA, Arab A, Wai EK. Effect of perioperative vitamin C supplementation on postoperative pain and the incidence of chronic regional pain syndrome: a systematic review and meta-analysis. *Clinical Journal of Pain* 2016; 32: 179-185. doi: 10.1097/AJP.0000000000000218

De Oliveira GS Jr, Castro-Alves LJ, Khan JH, McCarthy RJ. Perioperative systemic magnesium to minimize postoperative pain: a meta-analysis of randomized controlled trials. *Anesthesiology* 2013; 119: 178-190. doi: 10.1097/aln.0b013e318297630d.

Derry CJ, Derry S, Moore RA. Caffeine as an analgesic adjuvant for acute pain in adults. *Cochrane Database of Systematic Reviews* 2014; CD009281. doi: 10.1002/14651858.cd009281.pub3.

Derry S, Rice AS, Cole P, Tan T, Moore RA. Topical capsaicin (high concentration) for chronic neuropathic pain in adults. *Cochrane Database of Systematic Reviews* 2017: CD007393. doi: 10.1002/14651858.cd007393.pub4

Di Giuseppe D, Crippa A, Orsini N, Wolk A. Fish consumption and risk of rheumatoid arthritis: a dose-response meta-analysis. *Arthritis Research & Therapy* 2014; 16: 446. doi: 10.1186/s13075-014-0446-8.

D'Mello C, Ronaghan N, Zaheer R, Dicay M, Le T, MacNaughton WK, Surrette MG, Swain MG. Probiotics improve inflammation-associated sickness behavior by altering communication

between the peripheral immune system and the brain. *Journal of Neuroscience* 2015: 35: 10821-10830.
doi: 10.1523/jneurosci.0575-15.2015.

Eke-Okoro UJ, Raffa RB, Pergolizzi JV Jr, Breve F, Taylor R Jr; NEMA Research Group. Curcumin in turmeric: Basic and clinical evidence for a potential role in analgesia. *Journal of Clinical Pharmacy and Therapeutics* 2018; 43: 460-466. doi: 10.1111/jcpt.12703.

Gagnier JJ, Oltean H, van Tulder MW, Berman BM, Bombardier C, Robbins CB. Herbal medicine for low back pain: A Cochrane review. *Spine* (Phila Pa 1976) 2016; 41: 116-133.
doi: 10.1097/brs.0000000000001310.

Goldberg RJ, Katz J. A meta-analysis of the analgesic effects of omega-3 polyunsaturated fatty acid supplementation for inflammatory joint pain. *Pain* 2007; 129: 210-223. doi: 10.1016/j.pain.2007.01.020

Guida F, Boccella S, Belardo C, Iannotta M, Piscitelli F, De Filippis F, Paino S, Ricciardi F, Siniscalco D, Marabese I, Luongo L, Ercolini D, Di Marzo V, Maione S. Altered gut microbiota and endocannabinoid system tone in vitamin D deficiency-mediated chronic pain. *Brain, Behavior, and Immunity* 2019 Apr 3.
doi: 10.1016/j.bbi.2019.04.006.

Kirkland AE, Sarlo GL, Holton KF. The role of magnesium in neurological disorders. *Nutrients* 2018; 10.
doi: 10.3390/nu10060730.

Kunnumakkara AB, Bordoloi D, Padmavathi G, Monisha J, Roy NK, Prasad S, Aggarwal BB. Curcumin, the golden nutraceutical: multitargeting for multiple chronic diseases. *British Journal of Pharmacology* 2017; 174: 1325-1348. doi: 10.1111/bph.13621.

Lakhan SE, Ford CT, Tepper D. Zingiberaceae extracts for pain: a systematic review and meta-analysis. *Nutrition Journal* 2015; 14: 50.
doi: 10.1186/s12937-015-0038-8.

Lipton RB, Diener HC, Robbins MS, Garas SY, Patel K. Caffeine in the management of patients with headache. *Journal of Headache and Pain* 2017; 18: 107. doi: 10.1186/s10194-017-0806-2.

Magnusson KR, Hauck L, Jeffrey BM, Elias V, Humphrey A, Nath R, Perrone A, Bermudez LE. Relationships between diet-related changes in the gut microbiome and cognitive flexibility. *Neuroscience* 2015; 300: 128–140.
doi: 10.1016/j.neuroscience.2015.05.016.

Mayer EA, Knight R, Mazmanian SK, Cryan JF, Tillisch K. Gut microbes and the brain: paradigm shift in neuroscience. *Journal of Neuroscience* 2014; 34: 15490-15496.
doi: 10.1523/jneurosci.3299-14.2014.

Ng QX, Koh SSH, Chan HW, Ho CYX. Clinical use of curcumin in depression: a meta-analysis. *Journal of the American Medical Directors Association* 2017; 18: 503-508.
doi: 10.1016/j.jamda.2016.12.071.

Ooi SL, Correa D, Pak SC. Probiotics, prebiotics, and low FODMAP diet for irritable bowel syndrome – What is the current evidence? *Complementary Therapies in Medicine* 2019; 43: 73-80.
doi: 10.1016/j.ctim.2019.01.010.

Orr SL. Diet and nutraceutical interventions for headache management: a review of the evidence. *Cephalalgia* 2016; 36: 1112-1133.
doi: 10.1177/0333102415590239

Peng YN, Sung FC, Huang ML, Lin CL, Kao CH. The use of intravenous magnesium sulfate on postoperative analgesia in orthopedic surgery: A systematic review of randomized controlled trials. *Medicine* (Baltimore) 2018; 97: e13583.
doi: 10.1097/md.0000000000013583.

Ramsden CE, Faurot KR, Zamora D, Suchindran CM, Macintosh BA, Gaylord S, Ringel A, Hibbeln JR, Feldstein AE, Mori TA, Barden A, Lynch C, Coble R, Mas E, Palsson O, Barrow DA, Mann JD. Targeted alteration of dietary n-3 and n-6 fatty acids for the treatment of chronic headaches: a randomized trial. *Pain* 2013; 154: 2441-2451. doi: 10.1016/j.pain.2013.07.028.

Roman P, Carrillo-Trabalón F, Sánchez-Labraca N, Cañadas F, Estévez AF, Cardona D. Are probiotic treatments useful on fibromyalgia syndrome or chronic fatigue syndrome patients? A systematic review. *Beneficial Microbes* 2018; 9: 603-611.
doi: 10.3920/bm2017.0125.

Scott JR, Hassett AL, Schrepf AD, Brummett CM, Harris RE, Clauw DJ, Harte SE. Moderate alcohol consumption is associated with reduced pain and fibromyalgia symptoms in chronic pain patients. *Pain Medicine* 2018; 19: 2515-2527. doi: 10.1093/pm/pny032.

Senftleber NK, Nielsen SM, Andersen JR, Bliddal H, Tarp S, Lauritzen L, Furst DE, Suarez-Almazor ME, Lyddiatt A, Christensen R. Marine oil supplements for arthritis pain: a systematic review and meta-analysis of randomized trials. *Nutrients* 2017; 9. doi: 10.3390/nu9010042.

Shibuya N, Humphers JM, Agarwal MR, Jupiter DC. Efficacy and safety of high-dose vitamin C on complex regional pain syndrome in extremity trauma and surgery--systematic review and meta-analysis. *Journal of Foot and Ankle Surgery* 2013; 52: 62-66. doi: 10.1053/j.jfas.2012.08.003.

Staudacher HM, Irving PM, Lomer MC, Whelan K. Mechanisms and efficacy of dietary FODMAP restriction in IBS. *Nature Reviews Gastroenterology & Hepatology* 2014; 11: 256–266. doi: 10.1038/nrgastro.2013.259.

Steenbergen L, Sellaro R, van Hemert S, Bosch JA, Colzato LS. A randomized controlled trial to test the effect of multispecies probiotics on cognitive reactivity to sad mood. *Brain, Behavior, and Immunity* 2015; 48: 258-264. doi: 10.1016/j.bbi.2015.04.003.

Straube S, Derry S, Straube C, Moore RA. Vitamin D for the treatment of chronic painful conditions in adults. *Cochrane Database of Systematic Reviews* 2015; cd007771.

Thompson DF, Saluja HS. Prophylaxis of migraine headaches with riboflavin: A systematic review. *Journal of Clinical Pharmacy and Therapeutics* 2017; 42: 394-403. doi: 10.1111/jcpt.12548.

Vaghef-Mehrabany E, Alipour B, Homayouni-Rad A, Sharif SK, Asghari-Jafarabadi M, Zavvari S. Probiotic supplementation improves inflammatory status in patients with rheumatoid arthritis. *Nutrition* 2014; 30: 430-435. doi: 10.1016/j.nut.2013.09.007.

van Hemert S, Breedveld AC, Rovers JM, Vermeiden JP, Witteman BJ, Smits MG, de Roos NM. Migraine associated with gastrointestinal disorders: review of the literature and clinical implications. *Frontiers in Neurology* 2014; 5: 241. doi: 10.3389/fneur.2014.00241.

Yousef AA, Al-deeb AE. A double-blinded randomised controlled study of the value of sequential intravenous and oral magnesium therapy in patients with chronic low back pain with a neuropathic component. *Anaesthesia* 2013; 68: 260-266. doi: 10.1111/anae.12107.

Chapter 8: Move that body

Bidonde J, Busch AJ, Webber SC, Schachter CL, Danyliw A, Overend TJ, Richards RS, Rader T. Aquatic exercise training for fibromyalgia. *Cochrane Database of Systematic Reviews* 2014: CD011336. doi: 10.1002/14651858.cd011336.

Busch AJ, Webber SC, Richards RS, Bidonde J, Schachter CL, Schafer LA, Danyliw A, Sawant A, Dal Bello-Haas V, Rader T, Overend TJ. Resistance exercise training for fibromyalgia. *Cochrane Database of Systematic Reviews* 2013; cd010884. doi: 10.1002/14651858.cd010884.

Chen YW, Hunt MA, Campbell KL, Peill K, Reid WD. The effect of Tai Chi on four chronic conditions – cancer, osteoarthritis, heart failure and chronic obstructive pulmonary disease: a systematic review and meta-analyses. *British Journal of Sports Medicine* 2016; 50: 397-407. doi: 10.1136/bjsports-2014-094388

Cohen EE, Ejsmond-Frey R, Knight N, Dunbar RI. Rowers' high: behavioural synchrony is correlated with elevated pain thresholds. *Biology Letters* 2010; 6: 106-108. doi: 10.1098/rsbl.2009.0670.

Fransen M, McConnell S, Harmer AR, Van der Esch M, Simic M, Bennell KL. Exercise for osteoarthritis of the knee. *Cochrane Database of Systematic Reviews* 2015: cd004376. doi: 10.1002/14651858.cd004376.pub3.

Geneen LJ, Moore RA, Clarke C, Martin D, Colvin LA, Smith BH. Physical activity and exercise for chronic pain in adults: an overview of Cochrane Reviews. *Cochrane Database of Systematic Reviews* 2017: cd011279. doi: 10.1002/14651858.cd011279.pub3.

Gross A, Kay TM, Paquin JP, Blanchette S, Lalonde P, Christie T, Dupont G, Graham N, Burnie SJ, Gelley G, Goldsmith CH, Forget M, Hoving JL, Brønfort G, Santaguida PL; Cervical Overview Group. Exercises for mechanical neck disorders. *Cochrane Database of Systematic Reviews* 2015: cd004250. doi: 10.1002/14651858.cd004250.pub5.

Hurley M, Dickson K, Hallett R, Grant R, Hauari H, Walsh N, Stansfield C, Oliver S. Exercise interventions and patient beliefs for people with hip, knee or hip and knee osteoarthritis: a mixed methods review. *Cochrane Database of Systematic Reviews* 2018: cd010842. doi: 10.1002/14651858.cd010842.pub2.

References

Jones MD, Booth J, Taylor JL, Barry BK. Aerobic training increases pain tolerance in healthy individuals. *Medicine & Science in Sports & Exercise* 2014; 46: 1640-1647. doi: 10.1249/mss.0000000000000273.

Kaleth AS, Slaven JE, Ang DC. Does increasing steps per day predict improvement in physical function and pain interference in adults with fibromyalgia? *Arthritis Care & Research* (Hoboken) 2014; 66: 1887-1894. doi: 10.1002/acr.22398.

Larsson A, Palstam A, Löfgren M, Ernberg M, Bjersing J, Bileviciute-Ljungar I, Gerdle B, Kosek E, Mannerkorpi K. Resistance exercise improves muscle strength, health status and pain intensity in fibromyalgia – a randomized controlled trial. *Arthritis Research & Therapy* 2015; 17: 161. doi: 10.1186/s13075-015-0679-1.

Lee AC, Harvey WF, Price LL, Han X, Driban JB, Iversen MD, Desai SA, Knopp HE, Wang C. Dose-response effects of tai chi and physical therapy exercise interventions in symptomatic knee osteoarthritis. PM&R: *The Journal of Injury, Function and Rehabilitation* 2018; 10: 712-723. doi: 10.1016/j.pmrj.2018.01.003.

Nijs J, Lluch Girbés E, Lundberg M, Malfliet A, Sterling M. Exercise therapy for chronic musculoskeletal pain: innovation by altering pain memories. *Manual Therapy* 2015; 20: 216-220. doi: 10.1016/j.math.2014.07.004.

O'Connor SR, Tully MA, Ryan B, Bleakley CM, Baxter GD, Bradley JM, McDonough SM. Walking exercise for chronic musculoskeletal pain: systematic review and meta-analysis. *Archives of Physical Medicine and Rehabilitation* 2015; 96: 724-734. doi: 10.1016/j.apmr.2014.12.003

Sluka KA, Frey-Law L, Hoeger Bement M. Exercise-induced pain and analgesia? Underlying mechanisms and clinical translation. *Pain* 2018; 159: S91-S97. doi: 10.1097/j.pain.0000000000001235.

Vaegter HB, Handberg G, Graven-Nielsen T. Isometric exercises reduce temporal summation of pressure pain in humans. *European Journal of Pain* 2015; 19: 973–983. doi: 10.1002/ejp.623.

Vanti C, Andreatta S, Borghi S, Guccione AA, Pillastrini P, Bertozzi L. The effectiveness of walking versus exercise on pain and function in chronic low back pain: a systematic review and meta-analysis of randomized trials. *Disability and Rehabilitation* 2019; 41: 622-632. doi: 10.1080/09638288.2017.1410730.

White DK, Tudor-Locke C, Zhang Y, Fielding R, LaValley M, Felson DT,

Gross KD, Nevitt MC, Lewis CE, Torner J, Neogi T. Daily walking and the risk of incident functional limitation in knee osteoarthritis: an observational study. *Arthritis Care & Research* 2014; 66: 1328-1336. doi: 10.1002/acr.22362.

Yamato TP, Maher CG, Saragiotto BT, Hancock MJ, Ostelo RW, Cabral CM, Menezes Costa LC, Costa LO. Pilates for low back pain. *Cochrane Database of Systematic Reviews* 2015: cd010265. doi: 10.1002/14651858.cd010265.pub2.

Yan JH, Gu WJ, Sun J, Zhang WX, Li BW, Pan L. Efficacy of Tai Chi on pain, stiffness and function in patients with osteoarthritis: a meta-analysis. *PLoS One* 2013; 8: e61672. doi: 10.1371/journal.pone.0061672.

Xiang Y, Lu L, Chen X, Wen Z. Does Tai Chi relieve fatigue? A systematic review and meta-analysis of randomized controlled trials. *PLoS One* 2017; 12: e0174872. doi: 10.1371/journal.pone.0174872.

Zou L, Sasaki JE, Wei GX, Huang T, Yeung AS, Neto OB, Chen KW, Hui SS. Effects of mind-body exercises (tai chi/yoga) on heart rate variability parameters and perceived stress: a systematic review with meta-analysis of randomized controlled trials. *Journal of Clinical Medicine* 2018; 7(11): pii: E404.. doi: 10.3390/jcm7110404.

Zou L, Zhang Y, Yang L, Loprinzi PD, Yeung AS, Kong J, Chen KW, Song W, Xiao T, Li H. Are mindful exercises safe and beneficial for treating chronic lower back pain? A systematic review and meta-analysis of randomized controlled trials. *Journal of Clinical Medicine* 2019; 8: 628. doi: 10.3390/jcm8050628.

Chapter 9: Experience the power of mindfulness

Bushnell MC, Case LK, Ceko M, Cotton VA, Gracely JL, Low LA, Pitcher MH, Villemure C. Effect of environment on the long-term consequences of chronic pain. *Pain* 2015; 156: S42-S49. doi: 10.1097/01.j.pain.0000460347.77341.bd.

Garland EL, Manusov EG, Froeliger B, Kelly A, Williams JM, Howard MO. Mindfulness-oriented recovery enhancement for chronic pain and prescription opioid misuse: Results from an early-stage randomized controlled trial. *Journal of Consulting and Clinical*

References

Psychology 2014; 82: 448-459. doi: 10.1037/a0035798.

Goyal M, Singh S, Sibinga EM, Gould NF, Rowland-Seymour A, Sharma R, Berger Z, Sleicher D, Maron DD, Shihab HM, Ranasinghe PD, Linn S, Saha S, Bass EB, Haythornthwaite JA. Meditation programs for psychological stress and well-being: A systematic review and meta-analysis. *JAMA Internal Medicine* 2014; 174: 357-368. doi: 10.1001/jamainternmed.2013.13018.

Hood MM, Jedel S. Mindfulness-based interventions in inflammatory bowel disease. *Gastroenterology Clinics of North America* 2017; 46: 859-874. doi: 10.1016/j.gtc.2017.08.008.

Jeitler M, Brunnhuber S, Meier L, Lüdtke R, Büssing A, Kessler C, Michalsen A. Effectiveness of Jyoti meditation for patients with chronic neck pain and psychological distress – a randomized controlled clinical trial. *The Journal of Pain* 2015; 16: 77. doi: 10.1016/j.jpain.2014.10.009.

Khoo EL, Small R, Cheng W, Hatchard T, Glynn B, Rice DB, Skidmore B, Kenny S, Hutton B, Poulin PA. Comparative evaluation of group-based mindfulness-based stress reduction and cognitive behavioural therapy for the treatment and management of chronic pain: A systematic review and network meta-analysis. *Evidence-Based Mental Health* 2019; 22: 26-35. doi: 10.1136/ebmental-2018-300062.

Lauche R, Cramer H, Dobos G, Langhorst J, Schmidt S. A systematic review and meta-analysis of mindfulness-based stress reduction for the fibromyalgia syndrome. *Journal of Psychosomatic Research* 2013; 75: 500-510. doi: 10.1016/j.jpsychores.2013.10.010.

Lorenc A, Feder G, MacPherson H, Little P, Mercer SW, Sharp D. Scoping review of systematic reviews of complementary medicine for musculoskeletal and mental health conditions. *BMJ Open* 2018; 8: e020222. doi: 10.1136/bmjopen-2017-020222.

Morgan N, Irwin MR, Chung M, Wang C. The effects of mind-body therapies on the immune system: meta-analysis. *PLoS One* 2014; 9: e100903. doi: 10.1371/journal.pone.0100903.

Nascimento SS, Oliveira LR, DeSantana JM. Correlations between brain changes and pain management after cognitive and meditative therapies: a systematic review of neuroimaging studies. *Complementary Therapies in Medicine* 2018; 39: 137-145. doi: 10.1016/j.ctim.2018.06.006.

Neilson K, Ftanou M, Monshat K, Salzberg M, Bell S, Kamm MA, Connell W, Knowles SR, Sevar K, Mancuso SG, Castle D. A controlled study of a group mindfulness intervention for individuals living with inflammatory bowel disease. *Inflammatory Bowel Diseases* 2016; 22: 694-701. doi: 10.1097/mib.0000000000000629.

Schutte NS, Malouff JM. A meta-analytic review of the effects of mindfulness meditation on telomerase activity. *Psychoneuroendocrinology* 2014; 42: 45-48. doi: 10.1016/j.psyneuen.2013.12.017.

Tang YY, Hölzel BK, Posner MI. The neuroscience of mindfulness meditation. *Nature Reviews Neuroscience* 2015; 16: 213-225. doi: 10.1038/nrn3916

Theadom A, Cropley M, Smith HE, Feigin VL, McPherson K. Mind and body therapy for fibromyalgia. *Cochrane Database of Systematic Reviews* 2015: cd001980. doi: 10.1002/14651858.cd001980.pub3.

Wang X, Li P, Pan C, Dai L, Wu Y, Deng Y. The effect of mind-body therapies on insomnia: A systematic review and meta-analysis. *Evidence-Based Complementary and Alternative Medicine* 2019; 2019: 9359807. doi: 10.1155/2019/9359807.

Zeidan F, Salomons T, Farris SR, Emerson NM, Adler-Neal A, Jung Y, Coghill RC. Neural mechanisms supporting the relationship between dispositional mindfulness and pain. *Pain* 2018; 159: 2477-2485. doi: 10.1097/j.pain.0000000000001344.

Chapter 10: Keep working – don't give up

Ask T, Skouen JS, Assmus J, Kvåle A. Self-reported and tested function in health care workers with musculoskeletal disorders on full, partial or not on sick leave. *Journal of Occupational Rehabilitation* 2015; 25: 506-17. doi: 10.1007/s10926-014-9557-y.

Brooks J, McCluskey S, King N, Burton K. Illness perceptions in the context of differing work participation outcomes: exploring the influence of significant others in persistent back pain. *BMC Musculoskeletal Disorders* 2013; 14: 48. doi: 10.1186/1471-2474-14-48.

Carriere JS, Thibault P, Adams H, Milioto M, Ditto B, Sullivan MJL. Expectancies mediate the relationship between perceived injustice and return to work following whiplash injury: a 1-year prospective study. *European Journal of Pain* 2017; 21: 1234-1242. doi: 10.1002/ejp.1023.

de Vries HJ, Reneman MF, Groothoff JW, Geertzen JH, Brouwer S. Workers who stay at work despite chronic nonspecific musculoskeletal pain: do they differ from workers with sick leave? *Journal of Occupational Rehabilitation* 2012; 22: 489-502. doi: 10.1007/s10926-012-9360-6.

de Vries HJ, Reneman MF, Groothoff JW, Geertzen JH, Brouwer S. Self-reported work ability and work performance in workers with chronic nonspecific musculoskeletal pain. *Journal of Occupational Rehabilitation* 2013; 23: 1-10. doi: 10.1007/s10926-012-9373-1.

de Wit M, Wind H, Hulshof CTJ, Frings-Dresen MHW. Person-related factors associated with work participation in employees with health problems: a systematic review. *International Archives of Occupational and Environmental Health* 2018; 91: 497-512. doi: 10.1007/s00420-018-1308-5.

Kausto J, Solovieva S, Virta LJ, Viikari-Juntura E. Partial sick leave associated with disability pension: propensity score approach in a register-based cohort study. *BMJ Open* 2012; 2: e001752. doi: 10.1136/bmjopen-2012-001752.

Lewis M, Wynne-Jones G, Barton P, Whitehurst DG, Wathall S, Foster NE, Hay EM, van der Windt D. Should general practitioners issue a sick certificate to employees who consult for low back pain in primary care? *Journal of Occupational Rehabilitation* 2015; 25: 577-588. doi: 10.1007/s10926-014-9564-z.

Roberts MH, Klatzkin RR, Mechlin B. Social support attenuates physiological stress responses and experimental pain sensitivity to cold pressor pain. *Annals of behavioral medicine* 2015; 49: 557-569. doi: 10.1007/s12160-015-9686-3.

Sabariego C, Coenen M, Ito E, Fheodoroff K, Scaratti C, Leonardi M, Vlachou A, Stavroussi P, Brecelj V, Kovačič DS, Esteban E. Effectiveness of integration and re-integration into work strategies for persons with chronic conditions: a systematic review of European strategies. *International Journal of Environmental Research and Public Health* 2018; 15. doi: 10.3390/ijerph15030552.

Snippen NC, de Vries HJ, van der Burg-Vermeulen SJ, Hagedoorn M, Brouwer S. Influence of significant others on work participation of individuals with chronic diseases: a systematic review. *BMJ Open* 2019; 9: e021742. doi: 10.1136/bmjopen-2018-021742.

Viikari-Juntura E, Kausto J, Shiri R, Kaila-Kangas L, Takala EP, Karppinen J, Miranda H, Luukkonen R, Martimo KP. Return to work after early part-time sick leave due to musculoskeletal disorders: a randomized controlled trial. *Scandinavian Journal of Work, Environment and Health* 2012; 38: 134-143. doi: 10.5271/sjweh.3258.

Viikari-Juntura E, Leinonen T, Virta LJ, Hiljanen I, Husgafvel-Pursiainen K, Autti-Rämö I, Rissanen P, Burdorf A, Solovieva S. Early part-time sick leave results in considerable savings in social security costs at national level: an analysis based on a quasi-experiment in Finland. *Scandinavian Journal of Work, Environment & Health* 2019; 45: 203-208. doi: 10.5271/sjweh.3780.

Wynne-Jones G, Cowen J, Jordan JL, Uthman O, Main CJ, Glozier N, van der Windt D. Absence from work and return to work in people with back pain: A systematic review and meta-analysis. *Occupational and Environmental Medicine* 2014; 71: 448-456. doi: 10.1136/oemed-2013-101571.

Zale EL, Lange KL, Fields SA, Ditre JW. The relation between pain-related fear and disability: A meta-analysis. *Journal of Pain* 2013; 14: 1019-1030. doi: 10.1016/j.jpain.2013.05.005

Chapter 11: Be open to love and affection

Burns JW, Peterson KM, Smith DA, Keefe FJ, Porter LS, Schuster E, Kinner E. Temporal associations between spouse criticism/hostility and pain among patients with chronic pain: A within-couple daily diary study. *Pain* 2013; 154: 2715–2721. doi: 10.1016/j.pain.2013.07.053.

Coan JA, Beckes L, Gonzalez MZ, Maresh EL, Brown CL, Hasselmo K. Relationship status and perceived support in the social regulation of neural responses to threat. *Social Cognitive and Affective Neuroscience* 2017; 12: 1574-1583. doi: 10.1093/scan/nsx091.

Elvemo NA, Landrø NI, Borchgrevink PC, Håberg AK. Reward responsiveness in patients with chronic pain. *European Journal of Pain* 2015; 19: 1537-1543. doi: 10.1002/ejp.687.

Gouin JP, Carter CS, Pournajafi-Nazarloo H, Glaser R, Malarkey WB,

References

Loving TJ, Stowell J, Kiecolt-Glaser JK. Marital behavior, oxytocin, vasopressin, and wound healing. *Psychoneuroendocrinology* 2010; 35: 1082–1090. doi: 10.1016/j.psyneuen.2010.01.009.

Heim C, Newport DJ, Mletzko T, Miller AH, Nemeroff CB. The link between childhood trauma and depression: insights from HPA axis studies in humans. *Psychoneuroendocrinology* 2008; 33: 693-710. doi: 10.1016/j.psyneuen.2008.03.008.

Hemphill RC, Martire LM, Polenick CA, Stephens MA. Spouse confidence and physical function among adults with osteoarthritis: The mediating role of spouse responses to pain. *Health Psychology* 2016; 35: 1059-1068. doi: 10.1037/hea0000383.

Hsu DT, Sanford BJ, Meyers KK, Love TM, Hazlett KE, Wang H, Ni L, Walker SJ, Mickey BJ, Korycinski ST, Koeppe RA, Crocker JK, Langenecker SA, Zubieta JK. Response of the µ-opioid system to social rejection and acceptance. *Molecular Psychiatry* 2013; 18: 1211-1217. doi: 10.1038/mp.2013.96.

Marazziti D, Canale D. Hormonal changes when falling in love. *Psychoneuroendocrinology* 2004; 29: 931-936.

Nilakantan A, Younger J, Aron A, Mackey S. Preoccupation in an early-romantic relationship predicts experimental pain relief. *Pain Medicine* 2014; 15: 947-953. doi: 10.1111/pme.12422

Pow J, Stephenson E, Hagedoorn M, DeLongis A. Spousal support for patients with rheumatoid arthritis: getting the wrong kind is a pain. *Frontiers in Psychology* 2018; 9: 1760. doi: 10.3389/fpsyg.2018.01760.

Reese JB, Somers TJ, Keefe FJ, Mosley-Williams A, Lumley MA. Pain and functioning of rheumatoid arthritis patients based on marital status: Is a distressed marriage preferable to no marriage? *Journal of Pain* 2010; 11: 958-964. doi: 10.1016/j.jpain.2010.01.003.

Taylor SS, Davis MC, Zautra AJ. Relationship status and quality moderate daily pain-related changes in physical disability, affect, and cognitions in women with chronic pain. *Pain* 2013; 154: 147–153. doi: 10.1016/j.pain.2012.10.004.

Tracy LM, Ioannou L, Baker KS, Gibson SJ, Georgiou-Karistianis N, Giummarra MJ. Meta-analytic evidence for decreased heart rate variability in chronic pain implicating parasympathetic nervous system dysregulation. *Pain* 2016; 157: 7-29. doi: 10.1097/j.pain.0000000000000360.

Von Korff M, Alonso J, Ormel J, Angermeyer M, Bruffaerts R, Fleiz C, de Girolamo G, Kessler RC, Kovess-Masfety V, Posada-Villa J, Scott KM, Uda H. Childhood psychosocial stressors and adult onset arthritis: broad spectrum risk factors and allostatic load. *Pain* 2009; 143: 76-83. doi: 10.1016/j.pain.2009.01.034.

von Mohr M, Krahé C, Beck B, Fotopoulou A. The social buffering of pain by affective touch: a laser-evoked potential study in romantic couples. *Social Cognitive and Affective Neuroscience* 2018; 13: 1121-1130. doi: 10.1093/scan/nsy085.

Younger J, Aron A, Parke S, Chatterjee N, Mackey S. Viewing pictures of a romantic partner reduces experimental pain: involvement of neural reward systems. *PLoS One* 2010; 5: e13309.
doi: 10.1371/journal.pone.0013309.

Chapter 12: Get a pet

Beetz A, Uvnäs-Moberg K, Julius H, Kotrschal K. Psychosocial and psychophysiological effects of human-animal interactions: The possible role of oxytocin. *Frontiers in Psychology* 2012; 3: 234.
doi: 10.3389/fpsyg.2012.00234.

Carr ECJ, Wallace JE, Pater R, Gross DP. Evaluating the relationship between well-being and living with a dog for people with chronic low back pain: a feasibility study. *International Journal of Environmental Research and Public Health* 2019; 16. doi: 10.3390/ijerph16081472.

Håkanson M, Möller M, Lindström I, Mattsson B. The horse as the healer – a study of riding in patients with back pain. *Journal of Bodywork and Movement Therapies* 2009; 13: 43-52.
doi: 10.1016/j.jbmt.2007.06.002.

Halm MA. The healing power of the human-animal connection. *American Journal of Critical Care* 2008; 17: 373–376.

Harper CM, Dong Y, Thornhill TS, Wright J, Ready J, Brick GW, Dyer G. Can therapy dogs improve pain and satisfaction after total joint arthroplasty? A randomized controlled trial. *Clinical Orthopaedics and Related Research* 2015; 473: 372-379.
doi: 10.1007/s11999-014-3931-0.

Havey J, Vlasses FR, Vlasses PH, Ludwig-Beymer, Hackbarth D. The effect of animal-assisted therapy on pain medication use after

joint replacement. *Anthrozoos: A Multidisciplinary Journal of The Interactions of People & Animals* 2014; 27: 3.
doi: 10.2752/175303714X13903827487962

Huber A, Barber ALA, Faragó T, Müller CA, Huber L. Investigating emotional contagion in dogs (Canis familiaris) to emotional sounds of humans and conspecifics. *Animal Cognition* 2017; 20: 703-715. doi: 10.1007/s10071-017-1092-8.

Kumpula Sari. Culture for pain – Case: cultural activation period in a closed Facebook group among Finnish Pain Association. Thesis for the Bachelor's degree in Applied Science (cultural management). Helsinki, Finland, 2015 (abstract in English).

Lundqvist M, Carlsson P, Sjödahl R, Theodorsson E, Levin LÅ. Patient benefit of dog-assisted interventions in health care: a systematic review. *BMC Complementary and Alternative Medicine* 2017; 17: 358. doi: 10.1186/s12906-017-1844-7.

Marcus DA, Bernstein CD, Constantin JM, Kunkel FA, Breuer P, Hanlon RB. Animal-assisted therapy at an outpatient pain management clinic. *Pain Medicine* 2012; 13: 45-57.
doi: 10.1111/j.1526-4637.2011.01294.x.

Marcus DA, Bernstein CD, Constantin JM, Kunkel FA, Breuer P, Hanlon RB. Impact of animal-assisted therapy for outpatients with fibromyalgia. *Pain Medicine* 2013; 14: 43–51.
doi: 10.1111/j.1526-4637.2012.01522.x.

Müller CA, Schmitt K, Barber AL, Huber L. Dogs can discriminate emotional expressions of human faces. *Current Biology* 2014; 25: 601–605. doi: 10.1016/j.cub.2014.12.055.

Nagasawa M, Mitsui S, En S, Ohtani N, Ohta M, Sakuma Y, Onaka T, Mogi K, Kikusui T. Social evolution. Oxytocin-gaze positive loop and the coevolution of human-dog bonds. *Science* 2015; 348: 333-336. doi: 10.1126/science.1261022

Chapter 13: Manage your weight

Calvin AD, Carter RE, Adachi T, Macedo PG, Albuquerque FN, van der Walt C, Bukartyk J, Davison DE, Levine JA, Somers VK. Effects of experimental sleep restriction on caloric intake and activity energy expenditure. *Chest* 2013; 144: 79-86. doi: 10.1378/chest.12-2829.

Choi KW, Somers TJ, Babyak MA, Sikkema KJ, Blumenthal JA, Keefe FJ. The relationship between pain and eating among overweight and obese individuals with osteoarthritis: an ecological momentary study. *Pain Research & Management: The Journal of the Canadian Pain Society* 2014; 19: e159-163.

Christensen R, Henriksen M, Leeds AR, Gudbergsen H, Christensen P, Sørensen TJ, Bartels EM, Riecke BF, Aaboe J, Frederiksen R, Boesen M, Lohmander LS, Astrup A, Bliddal H. Effect of weight maintenance on symptoms of knee osteoarthritis in obese patients: a twelve-month randomized controlled trial. *Arthritis Care and Research* 2015; 67: 640-650. doi: 10.1002/acr.22504.

Cooper L, Ryan CG, Ells LJ, Hamilton S, Atkinson G, Cooper K, Johnson MI, Kirwan JP, Martin D. Weight loss interventions for adults with overweight/obesity and chronic musculoskeletal pain: a mixed methods systematic review. *Obesity Reviews* 2018; 19: 989-1007. doi: 10.1111/obr.12686.

Dario AB, Ferreira ML, Refshauge KM, Lima TS, Ordoñana JR, Ferreira PH3. The relationship between obesity, low back pain, and lumbar disc degeneration when genetics and the environment are considered: a systematic review of twin studies. *Spine Journal* 2015; 15: 1106-1117. doi: 10.1016/j.spinee.2015.02.001.

Groen VA, van de Graaf VA, Scholtes VA, Sprague S, van Wagensveld BA, Poolman RW. Effects of bariatric surgery for knee complaints in (morbidly) obese adult patients: a systematic review. *Obesity Reviews* 2015; 16: 161-170. doi: 10.1111/obr.12236.

Hall M, Castelein B, Wittoek R, Calders P, Van Ginckel A. Diet-induced weight loss alone or combined with exercise in overweight or obese people with knee osteoarthritis: a systematic review and meta-analysis. *Seminars in Arthritis and Rheumatism* 2019; 48: 765-777. doi: 10.1016/j.semarthrit.2018.06.005.

Kakeda T, Ogino Y, Moriya F, Saito S. Sweet taste-induced analgesia: An fMRI study. *Neuroreport* 2010; 21: 427-431. doi: 10.1097/WNR.0b013e3283383df5.

Karlsson HK, Tuominen L, Tuulari JJ, Hirvonen J, Parkkola R, Helin S, Salminen P, Nuutila P, Nummenmaa L. Obesity is associated with decreased μ-opioid but unaltered dopamine D2 receptor availability in the brain. *Journal of Neuroscience* 2015; 35: 3959-3965. doi: 10.1523/jneurosci.4744-14.2015.

References

Khoueir P, Black MH, Crookes PF, Kaufman HS, Katkhouda N, Wang MY. Prospective assessment of axial back pain symptoms before and after bariatric weight reduction surgery. *Spine Journal* 2009; 9: 454-463. doi: 10.1016/j.spinee.2009.02.003

King WC, Chen JY, Belle SH, Courcoulas AP, Dakin GF, Flum DR, Hinojosa MW, Kalarchian MA, Mitchell JE, Pories WJ, Spaniolas K, Wolfe BM, Yanovski SZ, Engel SG, Steffen KJ. Use of prescribed opioids before and after bariatric surgery: prospective evidence from a U.S. multicenter cohort study. *Surgery for Obesity and Related Diseases* 2017; 13: 1337-1346. doi: 10.1016/j.soard.2017.04.003.

Lasikiewicz N, Myrissa K, Hoyland A, Lawton CL. Psychological benefits of weight loss following behavioural and/or dietary weight loss interventions. A systematic research review. *Appetite* 2014; 72: 123-137. doi: 10.1016/j.appet.2013.09.017.

Nummenmaa L, Saanijoki T, Tuominen L, Hirvonen J, Tuulari JJ, Nuutila P, Kalliokoski K. μ-opioid receptor system mediates reward processing in humans. *Nature Communications* 2018; 9: 1500. doi: 10.1038/s41467-018-03848-y.

Okifuji A, Hare BD. The association between chronic pain and obesity. *Journal of Pain Research* 2015; 8: 399-408. doi: 10.2147/JPR.S55598.

Parent MB, Darling JN, Henderson YO. Remembering to eat: Hippocampal regulation of meal onset. *American Journal of Physiology – Regulatory, Integrative and Comparative Physiology* 2014; 306: r701-713. doi: 10.1152/ajpregu.00496.2013.

Raebel MA, Newcomer SR, Reifler LM, Boudreau D, Elliott TE, DeBar L, Ahmed A, Pawloski PA, Fisher D, Donahoo WT, Bayliss EA. Chronic use of opioid medications before and after bariatric surgery. *Journal of the American Medical Association* 2013; 310: 1369-1376. doi: 10.1001/jama.2013.278344.

Shin H, Shin J, Liu PY, Dutton GR, Abood DA, Ilich JZ. Self-efficacy improves weight loss in overweight/obese postmenopausal women during a 6-month weight loss intervention. *Nutrition Research* 2011; 31: 822-828. doi: 10.1016/j.nutres.2011.09.022.

Teixeira PJ, Carraça EV, Marques MM, Rutter H, Oppert JM, De Bourdeaudhuij I, Lakerveld J, Brug J. Successful behavior change in obesity interventions in adults: A systematic review of self-regulation mediators. *BMC Medicine* 2015; 13: 84. doi: 10.1186/s12916-015-0323-6.

Chapter 14: Give up smoking

Aimer P, Stamp L, Stebbings S, Valentino N, Cameron V, Treharne GJ. Identifying barriers to smoking cessation in rheumatoid arthritis. *Arthritis Care & Research* (Hoboken) 2015; 67: 607-615. doi: 10.1002/acr.22503

Behrend C, Prasarn M, Coyne E, Horodyski M, Wright J, Rechtine GR. Smoking cessation related to improved patient-reported pain scores following spinal care. *The Journal of Bone and Joint Surgery, American volume* 2012; 94: 2161-2166. doi: 10.2106/jbjs.k.01598

Bishop JY, Santiago-Torres JE, Rimmke N, Flanigan DC. Smoking predisposes to rotator cuff pathology and shoulder dysfunction: a systematic review. *Arthroscopy* 2015; 31: 1598-1605. doi: 10.1016/j.arthro.2015.01.026.

Hooten WM, Shi Y, Gazelka HM, Warner DO. The effects of depression and smoking on pain severity and opioid use in patients with chronic pain. *Pain* 2011; 152: 223-229. doi: 10.1016/j.pain.2010.10.045.

Kosiba JD, Zale EL, Ditre JW. Associations between pain intensity and urge to smoke: testing the role of negative affect and pain catastrophizing. *Drug and Alcohol Dependence* 2018; 187: 100-108. doi: 10.1016/j.drugalcdep.2018.01.037.

Martin LM, Sayette MA. A review of the effects of nicotine on social functioning. *Experimental and Clinical Psychopharmacology* 2018; 26: 425-439. doi: 10.1037/pha0000208.

Petre B, Torbey S, Griffith JW, De Oliveira G, Herrmann K, Mansour A, Baria AT, Baliki MN, Schnitzer TJ, Apkarian AV. Smoking increases risk of pain chronification through shared corticostriatal circuitry. *Human Brain Mapping* 2015: 36: 683–694. doi: 10.1002/hbm.22656.

Rajabi A, Dehghani M, Shojaei A, Farjam M, Motevalian SA. Association between tobacco smoking and opioid use: A meta-analysis. *Addictive Behaviors* 2019; 92: 225-235. doi: 10.1016/j.addbeh.2018.11.043.

Secades-Villa R, González-Roz A, García-Pérez Á, Becoña E. Psychological, pharmacological, and combined smoking cessation interventions for smokers with current depression: a systematic review and meta-analysis. *PLoS One* 2017; 12: e0188849.

doi: 10.1371/journal.pone.0188849.

Taylor G, McNeill A, Girling A, Farley A, Lindson-Hawley N, Aveyard P. Change in mental health after smoking cessation: Systematic review and meta-analysis. *British Medical Journal BMJ* 2014; 348. doi: 10.1136/bmj.g1151.

Chapter 15: Try yoga

Aboagye E, Karlsson ML, Hagberg J, Jensen I. Cost-effectiveness of early interventions for non-specific low back pain: A randomized controlled study investigating medical yoga, exercise therapy and self-care advice. *Journal of Rehabilitation in Medicine* 2015; 47: 167-173. doi: 10.2340/16501977-1910.

Bravo C, Skjaerven LH, Guitard Sein-Echaluce L, Catalan-Matamoros D. Effectiveness of movement and body awareness therapies in patients with fibromyalgia: a systematic review and meta-analysis. *European Journal of Physical and Rehabilitation Medicine* 2019 May 15. doi: 10.23736/S1973-9087.19.05291-2.

Bushnell MC, Case LK, Ceko M, Cotton VA, Gracely JL, Low LA, Pitcher MH, Villemure C. Effect of environment on the long-term consequences of chronic pain. *Pain* 2015; 156: S42-S49. doi: 10.1097/01.j.pain.0000460347.77341.bd.

Cramer H, Anheyer D, Lauche R, Dobos G. A systematic review of yoga for major depressive disorder. *Journal of Affective Disorders* 2017; 213: 70-77. doi: 10.1016/j.jad.2017.02.006.

Cramer H, Lauche R, Anheyer D, Pilkington K, de Manincor M, Dobos G, Ward L. Yoga for anxiety: a systematic review and meta-analysis of randomized controlled trials. *Depression and Anxiety* 2018; 35: 830-843. doi: 10.1002/da.22762.

Danhauer SC, Addington EL, Cohen L, Sohl SJ, Van Puymbroeck M, Albinati NK, Culos-Reed SN. Yoga for symptom management in oncology: A review of the evidence base and future directions for research. *Cancer* 2019; 125: 1979-1989. doi: 10.1002/cncr.31979.

Hartfiel N, Clarke G, Havenhand J, Phillips C, Edwards RT. Cost-effectiveness of yoga for managing musculoskeletal conditions in the workplace. *Occupational Medicine (London)* 2017; 67: 687-695. doi: 10.1093/occmed/kqx161.

Hernández SE, Barros-Loscertales A, Xiao Y, González-Mora JL, Rubia K. Gray matter and functional connectivity in anterior cingulate cortex are associated with the state of mental silence during Sahaja Yoga meditation. *Neuroscience* 2018; 371: 395-406. doi: 10.1016/j.neuroscience.2017.12.017.

Lee C, Crawford C, Schoomaker E; Active Self-Care Therapies for Pain (PACT) Working Group. Movement therapies for the self-management of chronic pain symptoms. *Pain Medicine* 2014; 15: S40-S53. doi: 10.1111/pme.12411.

Millstine D, Chen CY, Bauer B. Complementary and integrative medicine in the management of headache. *BMJ* 2017; 357: j1805. doi: 10.1136/bmj.j1805.

Nahin RL, Boineau R, Khalsa PS, Stussman BJ, Weber WJ. Evidence-based evaluation of complementary health approaches for pain management in the United States. *Mayo Clinic Proceedings* 2016; 91: 1292-1306. doi: 10.1016/j.mayocp.2016.06.007.

Oka T, Tanahashi T, Chijiwa T, Lkhagvasuren B, Sudo N, Oka K. Isometric yoga improves the fatigue and pain of patients with chronic fatigue syndrome who are resistant to conventional therapy: a randomized, controlled trial. *Biopsychosocial Medicine* 2014; 8: 27. doi: 10.1186/s13030-014-0027-8.

Wang Y, Lu S, Wang R, Jiang P, Rao F, Wang B, Zhu Y, Hu Y, Zhu J. Integrative effect of yoga practice in patients with knee arthritis: A PRISMA-compliant meta-analysis. *Medicine (Baltimore)* 2018; 97: e11742. doi: 10.1097/MD.0000000000011742.

Wells RE, Beuthin J, Granetzke L. Complementary and integrative medicine for episodic migraine: an update of evidence from the last 3 years. *Current Pain and Headache Reports* 2019; 23: 10. doi: 10.1007/s11916-019-0750-8.

Wieland LS, Skoetz N, Pilkington K, Vempati R, D'Adamo CR, Berman BM. Yoga treatment for chronic non-specific low back pain. *Cochrane Database of Systematic Reviews* 2017; cd010671. doi: 10.1002/14651858.cd010671.pub2.

Wren AA, Wright MA, Carson JW, Keefe FJ. Yoga for persistent pain: new findings and directions for an ancient practice. *Pain* 2011; 152: 477-480. doi: 10.1016/j.pain.2010.11.017.

Chapter 16: Try acupuncture

Baeumler PI, Fleckenstein J, Takayama S, Simang M, Seki T, Irnich D. Effects of acupuncture on sensory perception: A systematic review and meta-analysis. *PLoS One* 2014; 9: e113731. doi: 10.1371/journal.pone.0113731.

Cai RL, Shen GM, Wang H, Guan YY. Brain functional connectivity network studies of acupuncture: a systematic review on resting-state fMRI. *Journal of Integrative Medicine* 2018; 16: 26-33. doi: 10.1016/j.joim.2017.12.002.

Chae Y, Chang DS, Lee SH, Jung WM, Lee IS, Jackson S, Kong J, Lee H, Park HJ, Lee H, Wallraven C. Inserting needles into the body: a meta-analysis of brain activity associated with acupuncture needle stimulation. *Journal of Pain* 2013; 14: 215-222. doi: 10.1016/j.jpain.2012.11.011.

Hopton A, Macpherson H, Keding A, Morley S. Acupuncture, counselling or usual care for depression and comorbid pain: Secondary analysis of a randomised controlled trial. *BMJ Open* 2014; 4: e004964. doi: 10.1136/bmjopen-2014-004964.

Huang W, Pach D, Napadow V, Park K, Long X, Neumann J, Maeda Y, Nierhaus T, Liang F, Witt CM. Characterizing acupuncture stimuli using brain imaging with FMRI: a systematic review and meta-analysis of the literature. *PLoS One* 2012; 7: e32960. doi: 10.1371/journal.pone.0032960.

Karatay S, Okur SC, Uzkeser H, Yildirim K, Akcay F. Effects of acupuncture treatment on fibromyalgia symptoms, serotonin, and substance P levels: a randomized sham and placebo-controlled clinical trial. *Pain Medicine* 2018; 19: 615-628. doi: 10.1093/pm/pnx263.

Lai HC, Lin YW, Hsieh CL. Acupuncture-analgesia-mediated alleviation of central sensitization. *Evidence-Based Complementary and Alternative Medicine* 2019; 2019: 6173412. doi: 10.1155/2019/6173412.

Liu L, Skinner M, McDonough S, Mabire L, Baxter GD. Acupuncture for low back pain: an overview of systematic reviews. *Evidence-Based Complementary and Alternative Medicine* 2015: 328196. doi: 10.1155/2015/328196.

MacPherson H, Vertosick EA, Foster NE, Lewith G, Linde K, Sherman KJ, Witt CM, Vickers AJ. The persistence of the effects of acupuncture after a course of treatment: a meta-analysis of patients with chronic pain. *Pain* 2017; 158: 784-793. doi: 10.1097/j.pain.0000000000000747.

Vickers AJ, Vertosick EA, Lewith G, MacPherson H, Foster NE, Sherman KJ, Irnich D, Witt CM, Linde K; Acupuncture Trialists' Collaboration. Acupuncture for chronic pain: update of an individual patient data meta-analysis. *Journal of Pain* 2018; 19: 455-474. doi: 10.1016/j.jpain.2017.11.005.

Zhang XC, Chen H, Xu WT, Song YY, Gu YH, Ni GX. Acupuncture therapy for fibromyalgia: a systematic review and meta-analysis of randomized controlled trials. *Journal of Pain Research* 2019; 12: 527-542. doi: 10.2147/JPR.S186227.

Chapter 17: Be creative

Aalbers S, Fusar-Poli L, Freeman RE, Spreen M, Ket JC, Vink AC, Maratos A, Crawford M, Chen XJ, Gold C. Music therapy for depression. *Cochrane Database of Systematic Reviews* 2017; 11: cd004517. doi: 10.1002/14651858.cd004517.pub3.

Angheluta A-M, Lee BK. Art therapy for chronic pain: applications and future directions. *Canadian Journal of Counselling and Psychotherapy* 2011; 45: 112-131.

Archer S, Buxton S, Sheffield D. The effect of creative psychological interventions on psychological outcomes for adult cancer patients: A systematic review of randomised controlled trials. *Psycho-Oncology* 2015; 24: 1. doi: 10.1002/pon.3607.

Cheong YC, Smotra G, Williams AC. Non-surgical interventions for the management of chronic pelvic pain. *Cochrane Database of Systematic Reviews* 2014; cd008797. doi: 10.1002/14651858.cd008797.pub2.

Dobek CE, Beynon ME, Bosma RL, Stroman PW. Music modulation of pain perception and pain-related activity in the brain, brain stem, and spinal cord: a functional magnetic resonance imaging study. *Journal of Pain* 2014; 15: 1057-1068. doi: 10.1016/j.jpain.2014.07.006.

Dunbar RI, Kaskatis K, MacDonald I, Barra V. Performance of music elevates pain threshold and positive affect: implications for the evolutionary function of music. *Evolutionary Psychology* 2012; 10: 688-702.

Fancourt D, Steptoe A. Physical and psychosocial factors in the prevention of chronic pain in older age. *Journal of Pain* 2018; 19: 1385-1391. doi: 10.1016/j.jpain.2018.06.001.

Fritz TH, Bowling DL, Contier O, Grant J, Schneider L, Lederer A, Höer F, Busch E, Villringer A. Musical agency during physical exercise decreases pain. *Frontiers in Psychology* 2018; 8: 2312. doi: 10.3389/fpsyg.2017.02312.

Garza-Villarreal EA, Wilson AD, Vase L, Brattico E, Barrios FA, Jensen TS, Romero-Romo JI, Vuust P. Music reduces pain and increases functional mobility in fibromyalgia. *Frontiers in Psychology* 2014; 5: 90. doi: 10.3389/fpsyg.2014.00090.

Garza-Villarreal EA, Pando V, Vuust P, Parsons C. Music-induced analgesia in chronic pain conditions: a systematic review and meta-analysis. *Pain Physician* 2017; 20: 597-610.

Gramaglia C, Gambaro E, Vecchi C, Licandro D, Raina G, Pisani C, Burgio V, Farruggio S, Rolla R, Deantonio L, Grossini E, Krengli M, Zeppegno P. Outcomes of music therapy interventions in cancer patients – a review of the literature. *Critical Reviews in Oncology/Hematology* 2019; 138: 241-254. doi: 10.1016/j.critrevonc.2019.04.004.

Hole J, Hirsch M, Ball E, Meads C. Music as an aid for postoperative recovery in adults: a systematic review and meta-analysis. *Lancet* 2015; 386: 1659–1671. doi: 10.1016/S0140-6736(15)60169-6.

Karkou V, Aithal S, Zubala A, Meekums B. Effectiveness of dance movement therapy in the treatment of adults with depression: a systematic review with meta-analyses. *Frontiers in Psychology* 2019; 10: 936. doi: 10.3389/fpsyg.2019.00936.

Kelly CG, Cudney S, Weinert C. Use of creative arts as a complementary therapy by rural women coping with chronic illness. *Journal of Holistic Nursing* 2012; 30: 48-54. doi: 10.1177/0898010111423418.

Lee JH. The effects of music on pain: a review of systematic reviews and meta-analysis. Doctoral dissertation. University of Eastern Finland, Finland, 2012.

Loggia ML, Berna C, Kim J, Cahalan CM, Gollub RL, Wasan AD, Harris RE, Edwards RR, Napadow V. Disrupted brain circuitry for pain-related reward/punishment in fibromyalgia. *Arthritis and Rheumatology* 2014; 66: 203-212. doi: 10.1002/art.38191.

Martin-Saavedra JS, Vergara-Mendez LD, Talero-Gutiérrez C. Music is an effective intervention for the management of pain: an umbrella review. *Complementary Therapies in Clinical Practice* 2018; 32: 103-114. doi: 10.1016/j.ctcp.2018.06.003.

Maujean A, Pepping CA, Kendall E. A systematic review of randomized controlled studies of art therapy. *Art Therapy* 2014; 31: 37. doi.org/10.1080/07421656.2014.873696

Murillo-García Á, Villafaina S, Adsuar JC, Gusi N, Collado-Mateo D. Effects of dance on pain in patients with fibromyalgia: a systematic review and meta-analysis. *Evidence-Based Complementary and Alternative Medicine* 2018; 2018: 8709748. doi: 10.1155/2018/8709748.

Nightingale, F. *Notes on nursing: What it is and what it is not.* New York, US: D. Appleton and Company; 1860.

O'Neill M. Cultural attendance and public mental health – from research to practice. *Journal of Public Mental Health* 2010; 9: 22-29. doi: 10.5042/jpmh.2010.0700.

Stuckey HL, Nobel J. The connection between art, healing, and public health: A review of current literature. *American Journal of Public Health* 2010; 100: 254-263. doi: 10.2105/ajph.2008.156497.

Sunitha Suresh BS, De Oliveira GS Jr, Suresh S. The effect of audio therapy to treat postoperative pain in children undergoing major surgery: a randomized controlled trial. *Pediatric Surgery International* 2015; 31: 197-201. doi: 10.1007/s00383-014-3649-9.

Teixeira-Machado L, Arida RM, de Jesus Mari J. Dance for neuroplasticity: a descriptive systematic review. *Neuroscience & Biobehavioral Reviews* 2019; 96: 232-240. doi: 10.1016/j.neubiorev.2018.12.010.

Uttley L, Stevenson M, Scope A, Rawdin A, Sutton A. The clinical and cost effectiveness of group art therapy for people with non-psychotic mental health disorders: a systematic review and cost-effectiveness analysis. *BMC Psychiatry* 2015; 15: 151. doi: 10.1186/s12888-015-0528-4.

Vaajoki A. Postoperative pain in adult gastroenterological patients music intervention in pain alleviation. Doctoral dissertation. University of Eastern Finland, Finland, 2012.

Chapter 18: Consider medication

Berna C, Kulich RJ, Rathmell JP. Tapering long-term opioid therapy in chronic noncancer pain: evidence and recommendations for everyday practice. *Mayo Clinic Proceedings* 2015; 90: 828-842. doi: 10.1016/j.mayocp.2015.04.003.

Bostick GP, Toth C, Carr EC, Stitt LW, Morley-Forster P, Clark AJ, Lynch M, Gordon A, Nathan H, Smyth C, Ware MA, Moulin DE. Physical functioning and opioid use in patients with neuropathic pain. *Pain Medicine* 2015; 16: 1361-1368. doi: 10.1111/pme.12702.

Caruso R, Ostuzzi G, Turrini G, Ballette F, Recla E, Dall'Olio R, Croce E, Casoni B, Grassi L, Barbui C. Beyond pain: can antidepressants improve depressive symptoms and quality of life in patients with neuropathic pain? A systematic review and meta-analysis. *Pain* 2019 May 22. doi: 10.1097/j.pain.0000000000001622.

Clauw DJ. Fibromyalgia and related conditions. *Mayo Clinic Proceedings* 2015; 90: 680–692. doi: 10.1016/j.mayocp.2015.03.014.

de Zanette SA, Vercelino R, Laste G, Rozisky JR, Schwertner A, Machado CB, Xavier F, de Souza IC, Deitos A, Torres IL, Caumo W. Melatonin analgesia is associated with improvement of the descending endogenous pain-modulating system in fibromyalgia: a phase II, randomized, double-dummy, controlled trial. *BMC Pharmacology and Toxicology* 2014; 15: 40. doi: 10.1186/2050-6511-15-40.

Derry S, Bell RF, Straube S, Wiffen PJ, Aldington D, Moore RA. Pregabalin for neuropathic pain in adults. *Cochrane Database of Systematic Reviews* 2019; cd007076. doi: 10.1002/14651858.cd007076.pub3.

Derry S, Wiffen PJ, Häuser W, Mücke M, Tölle TR, Bell RF, Moore RA. Oral nonsteroidal anti-inflammatory drugs for fibromyalgia in adults. *Cochrane Database of Systematic Reviews* 2017; cd012332. doi: 10.1002/14651858.cd012332.pub2.

Derry S, Wiffen PJ, Kalso EA, Bell RF, Aldington D, Phillips T, Gaskell H, Moore RA. Topical analgesics for acute and chronic pain in adults – an overview of Cochrane Reviews. *Cochrane Database of Systematic Reviews* 2017: cd008609. doi: 10.1002/14651858.cd008609.pub2.

Dublin S, Walker RL, Gray SL, Hubbard RA, Anderson ML, Yu O, Crane PK, Larson EB. Prescription opioids and risk of dementia or cognitive decline: a prospective cohort study. *Journal of the American Geriatrics Society* 2015; 63: 1519–1526. doi: 10.1111/jgs.13562.

Eriksen J, Sjøgren P, Bruera E, Ekholm O, Rasmussen NK. Critical issues on opioids in chronic non-cancer pain: An epidemiological study. *Pain* 2006; 125: 172–179. doi: 10.1016/j.pain.2006.06.009

Finnerup NB, Attal N, Haroutounian S, McNicol E, Baron R, Dworkin RH, Gilron I, Haanpää M, Hansson P, Jensen TS, Kamerman PR, Lund K, Moore A, Raja SN, Rice AS, Rowbotham M, Sena E, Siddall P, Smith BH, Wallace M. Pharmacotherapy for neuropathic pain in adults: a systematic review and meta-analysis. *Lancet Neurology* 2015; 14: 162-173. doi: 10.1016/S1474-4422(14)70251-0.

Garland EL, Froeliger B, Zeidan F, Partin K, Howard MO. The downward spiral of chronic pain, prescription opioid misuse, and addiction: Cognitive, affective, and neuropsychopharmacologic pathways. *Neuroscience and Biobehavioral Reviews* 2013; 37: 2597-2607. doi: 10.1016/j.neubiorev.2013.08.006

Goesling J, Henry MJ, Moser SE, Rastogi M, Hassett AL, Clauw DJ, Brummett CM. Symptoms of depression are associated with opioid use regardless of pain severity and physical functioning among treatment-seeking patients with chronic pain. *Journal of Pain* 2015; 16: 844-851. doi: 10.1016/j.jpain.2015.05.010.

Halladin NL, Rosenberg J, Gögenur I, Møller AM, Hansen MV. Melatonin for pre- and postoperative anxiety in adults. *Cochrane Database of Systematic Reviews* 2015; cd009861. doi: 10.1002/14651858.cd009861.pub2

Hartwell EE, Pfeifer JG, McCauley JL, Moran-Santa Maria M, Back SE. Sleep disturbances and pain among individuals with prescription opioid dependence. *Addictive Behaviors* 2014; 39: 1537-1542. doi: 10.1016/j.addbeh.2014.05.025.

Hepp Z, Bloudek LM, Varon SF. Systematic review of migraine prophylaxis adherence and persistence. *Journal of Managed Care Pharmacy* 2014; 20: 22-33. doi: 10.18553/jmcp.2014.20.1.22

Moulin DE, Clark AJ, Gordon A, Lynch M, Morley-Forster PK, Nathan H, Smyth C, Toth C, VanDenKerkhof E, Gilani A, Ware MA. Long-term outcome of the management of chronic neuropathic pain: a prospective observational study. *Journal of Pain* 2015; 16: 852-861. doi: 10.1016/j.jpain.2015.05.011.

Moulin Lalic S, Gisev N, Bell JS, Korhonen MJ, Ilomäki J. Predictors of persistent prescription opioid analgesic use among people without cancer in Australia. *British Journal of Clinical Pharmacology* 2018; 84: 1267-1278. doi: 10.1111/bcp.13556.

Murphy JL, Clark ME, Banou E. Opioid cessation and multidimensional outcomes after interdisciplinary chronic pain treatment. *Clinical Journal of Pain* 2013; 29: 109-117. doi: 10.1097/ajp.0b013e3182579935.

Nijs J, Malfliet A, Ickmans K, Baert I, Meeus M. Treatment of central sensitization in patients with 'unexplained' chronic pain: an update. *Expert Opinion on Pharmacotherapy* 2014; 15: 1671-1683. doi: 10.1517/14656566.2014.925446.

Ong CK, Seymour RA, Lirk P, Merry AF. Combining paracetamol (acetaminophen) with nonsteroidal anti-inflammatory drugs: a qualitative systematic review of analgesic efficacy for acute postoperative pain. *Anesthesia and Analgesia* 2010; 110: 1170-1179. doi: 10.1213/ane.0b013e3181cf9281.

Peng X, Robinson RL, Mease P, Kroenke K, Williams DA, Chen Y, Faries D, Wohlreich M, McCarberg B, Hann D. Long-term evaluation of opioid treatment in fibromyalgia. *Clinical Journal of Pain* 2015; 31: 7-13. doi: 10.1097/ajp.0000000000000079.

Perrot S, Russell I. More ubiquitous effects from non-pharmacologic than from pharmacologic treatments for fibromyalgia syndrome: a meta-analysis examining six core symptoms. *European Journal of Pain* 2014; 18: 1067–1080. doi: 10.1002/ejp.564.

Raknes G, Småbrekke L. Low dose naltrexone: Effects on medication in rheumatoid and seropositive arthritis. A nationwide register-based controlled quasi-experimental before-after study. *PLoS One* 2019; 14: e0212460. doi: 10.1371/journal.pone.0212460

Ray WA, Chung CP, Murray KT, Hall K, Stein CM. Prescription of long-acting opioids and mortality in patients with chronic noncancer pain. *JAMA* 2016; 315: 2415-2423. doi: 10.1001/jama.2016.77

Robinson JP, Dansie EJ, Wilson HD, Rapp S, Turk DC. Attitudes and beliefs of working and work-disabled people with chronic pain prescribed long-term opioids. *Pain Medicine* 2015; 16: 1311-1324. doi: 10.1111/pme.12770.

Schwertner A, Conceição Dos Santos CC, Costa GD, Deitos A, de
    Souza A, de Souza IC, Torres IL, da Cunha Filho JS, Caumo W.
    Efficacy of melatonin in the treatment of endometriosis: a phase II,
    randomized, double-blind, placebo-controlled trial. *Pain* 2013; 154:
    874-881. doi: 10.1016/j.pain.2013.02.025.

Smith K, Mattick RP, Bruno R, Nielsen S, Cohen M, Campbell G,
    Larance B, Farrell M, Degenhardt L. Factors associated with the
    development of depression in chronic non-cancer pain patients
    following the onset of opioid treatment for pain. *Journal of Affective
    Disorders* 2015; 184: 72–80. doi: 10.1016/j.jad.2015.05.049.

Stefani LC, Muller S, Torres IL, Razzolini B, Rozisky JR, Fregni F,
    Markus R, Caumo W. A phase II, randomized, double-blind,
    placebo controlled, dose-response trial of the melatonin effect on
    the pain threshold of healthy subjects. *PLoS One* 2013; 8: e74107.
    doi: 10.1371/journal.pone.0074107.

Thorpe J, Shum B, Moore RA, Wiffen PJ, Gilron I. Combination
    pharmacotherapy for the treatment of fibromyalgia in adults.
    Cochrane Database of Systematic Reviews 2018: cd010585.
    doi: 10.1002/14651858.cd010585.pub2.

van Rijswijk SM, van Beek MHCT, Schoof GM, Schene AH, Steegers
    M, Schellekens AF. Iatrogenic opioid use disorder, chronic pain
    and psychiatric comorbidity: a systematic review. *General Hospital
    Psychiatry* 2019; 59: 37-50. doi: 10.1016/j.genhosppsych.2019.04.008.

Wasan AD, Michna E, Edwards RR, Katz JN, Nedeljkovic SS, Dolman
    AJ, Janfaza D, Isaac Z, Jamison RN. Psychiatric comorbidity is
    associated prospectively with diminished opioid analgesia and
    increased opioid misuse in patients with chronic low back pain.
    Anesthesiology 2015; 123: 861-872.
    doi: 10.1097/aln.0000000000000768.

Welsch P, Üçeyler N, Klose P, Walitt B, Häuser W. Serotonin and
    noradrenaline reuptake inhibitors (SNRIs) for fibromyalgia.
    Cochrane Database of Systematic Reviews 2018; CD010292.
    doi: 10.1002/14651858.CD010292.pub2.

Younger JW, Chu LF, D'Arcy NT, Trott KE, Jastrzab LE, Mackey SC.
    Prescription opioid analgesics rapidly change the human brain.
    Pain 2011; 152: 1803-1810. doi: 10.1016/j.pain.2011.03.028.

Younger J, Noor N, McCue R, Mackey S. Low-dose naltrexone for
    the treatment of fibromyalgia: findings of a small, randomized,

double-blind, placebo-controlled, counterbalanced, crossover trial assessing daily pain levels. *Arthritis & Rheumatology* 2013; 65: 529-538. doi: 10.1002/art.37734.

Younger J, Parkitny L, McLain D. The use of low-dose naltrexone (LDN) as a novel anti-inflammatory treatment for chronic pain. *Clinical Rheumatology* 2014; 33: 451-459. doi: 10.1007/s10067-014-2517-2.

Zeng C, Dubreuil M, LaRochelle MR, Lu N, Wei J, Choi HK, Lei G, Zhang Y. Association of tramadol with all-cause mortality among patients with osteoarthritis. *JAMA* 2019; 321: 969-982. doi: 10.1001/jama.2019.1347.

Zhu C, Xu Y, Duan Y, Li W, Zhang L, Huang Y, Zhao W, Wang Y, Li J, Feng T, Li X, Hu X, Yin W. Exogenous melatonin in the treatment of pain: a systematic review and meta-analysis. *Oncotarget* 2017; 8: 100582-100592. doi: 10.18632/oncotarget.21504.

Index

250

Index

Index

Index

Index